Glass House Books

Beating Drug Addiction in Tehran: A Women's Clinic

Dr Kate Dolan is a professor of public health at the University of New South Wales, Australia. She has carried out over 100 studies, has published over 270 publications and received $39 million in research funds. She has been a consultant for the International Narcotics Control Board, the United Nations and the World Health Organization. She received a Winston Churchill Fellowship to study managed alcohol programs. She received a Senior Fulbright Fellowship from Kansas State University to study solitary confinement in prison. She established the first methadone clinic for female drug users in Iran.

I0126377

GHB

Glass House Books
Brisbane

Glass House Books
an imprint of IP (Interactive Publications Pty Ltd)
Treetop Studio • 9 Kuhler Court
Carindale, Queensland, Australia 4152
sales@ipoz.biz
http://ipoz.biz/

Printed in 12 pt Adobe Caslon Pro on 14 pt Avenir Book.

ISBN: 9781922332325 (PB); 9781922332332 (eBk)

A catalogue record for this book is available from the National Library of Australia

The author's book *A cup of tea with abandoned angels: women using drugs in South Tehran,* The Contemporary Society, Tehran, 2016. (in Farsi) is available here

https://fidibo.com/book/66541 كتاب-كی-فنجان-چای-با-فرشتگان-راندە-شدە

Beating Drug Addiction in Tehran: a Women's Clinic

Professor Kate Dolan

GHB

Glass House Books
Brisbane

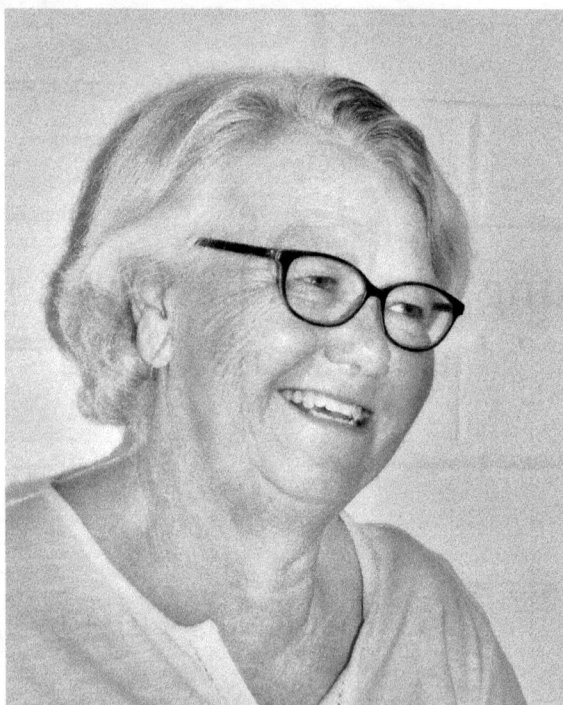

I dedicate this book to my parents Bill (deceased) and Mona who gave me so many opportunities and set my moral compass, and to my children Georgie and Billy, who I adore and cherish.

Acknowledgments

Author photo: Johanna Clifford
Book design: David P. Reiter

There are many people to acknowledge and thank for the establishment of the clinic and the conduct of the research that is the subject of my book. First I want to acknowledge all my colleagues in Tehran; the clinicians and researchers. I am forever indebted to Bijan who was already on this journey when I met him way back in 2002. His dedication to helping people who use drugs to have a better life was incredible. Next, I want to thank my hero, Parviz, his ground breaking work in the HIV field in prison was astounding. Roya was an amazing colleague who had my book translated and published in Farsi. There are many people who also were instrumental in assisting the clinic to come to fruition; Shabnam, Setareh, Azarakhsh, Gelareh and Fariba.

I also wish to acknowledge my Australian colleagues Alex, who found the funding, and David (now deceased), who assisted with data analyses.

Finally I want to thank the Drosos Foundation for funding the clinic and the research. And special thanks go to the women who came along to our clinic and trusted us with their health and shared their life stories.

Contents

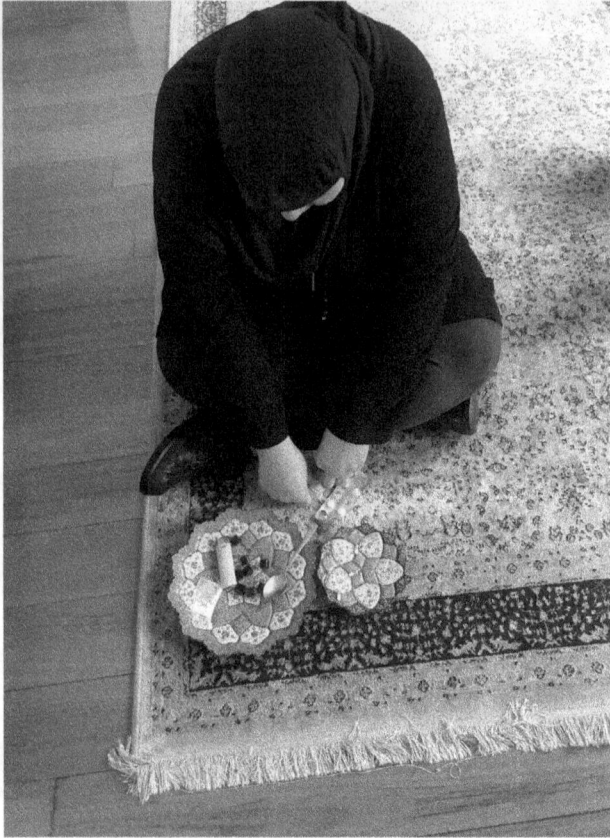

An Iranian woman preparing to inject drugs

Foreword

As an epidemiologist who has studied women who use drugs for decades, I have always wanted to accompany Kate Dolan on one of her trips to Iran for an insider's experience. *Beating Drug Addiction in Tehran* invites the reader to do just that, and it taught me more than I expected. Dolan draws from her vast international experience, weaving together the history and epidemiology of drug use in Iran with a tapestry of incredible, heart-rending stories from Iranian women experiencing the darkest depths of addiction. She chronicles her unflagging efforts to give these women a chance at recovery, but ends up giving them something more: dignity and respect. For readers who thought that epidemiologists were just 'bean counters', you're in for the shock of your lives.

Steffanie Strathdee, PhD
Associate Dean of Global Health Sciences,
Harold Simon Professor, UCSD Departmnt of Medicine
Co-Director, Center for Innovative Phage Applications and
Therapeutics https://ipath.ucsd.edu

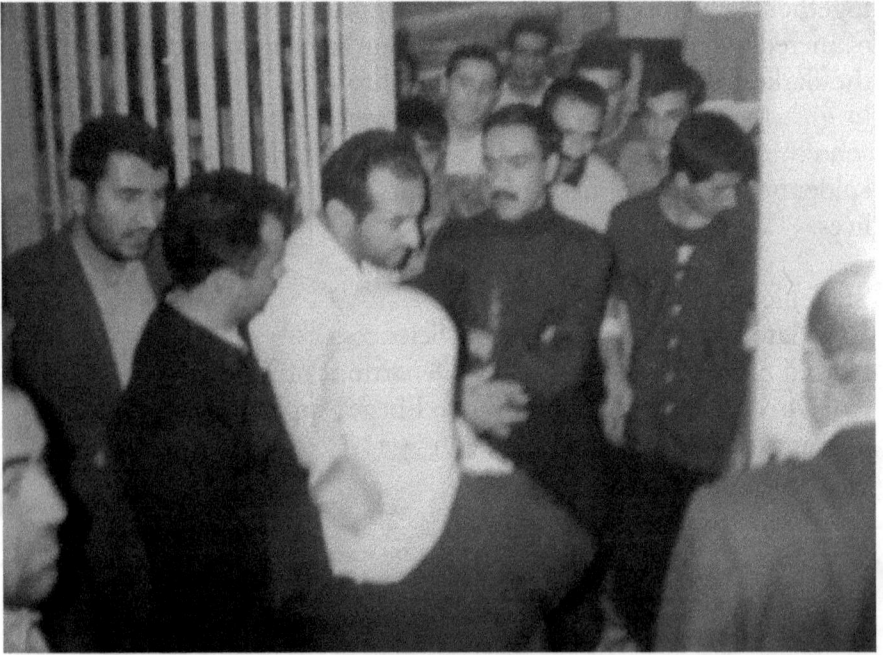

The author standing at the prison cell door where she met inmates

Chapter 1. Evin Prison

In 2003, I was invited to deliver training on HIV to prison doctors in Iran. After the training, I was taken on a study tour of Iranian prisons. When I asked about women in prison, I was offered a chance to tour their wing within Evin Prison. I had accepted immediately. This was an environment that we see and hear nothing of in the West. To enter the female wing, I had to walk through several metal doors from the male wing. Inside, the walls were white with a pale blue trim. I had just visited eight prisons for men over the last ten days. But it was this visit—to a female prison in Iran—which would have a lasting effect on me. It changed my focus at work, my circle of friends and the way I viewed Iran and Islam. This prison in North West Tehran was newish, having been built in 1971. It sat at the foot of the Alborz Mountains, which are covered in snow in winter. This was the first trip of many I would make to Iran over the next decade.

The foyer of the women's wing was clean like a hospital, sparse even. We walked down the corridor and there, on the right, was a cell. As we stood in the doorway, all the occupants turned away to hide, holding their chadors—long, flowing capes—up close under their chins. Each woman was wearing the same navy blue and white patterned chador, the prison-issue uniform. Some inmates had small children with them, and a few had babes in their arms. My visiting party comprised my interpreter, my guide, a prison guard and me.

Even with a borrowed hejab—the mandatory headscarf to cover a woman's hair—everyone could see I was a foreigner. Strands of my blonde hair protruded from my pale hejab and my peaches and cream complexion meant I was from somewhere other than Iran. The female inmates were taken aback, suspicious even, to see me, as were their male peers when I was in their prisons. The interpreter introduced us to the women. As the interpreter spoke, they slowly turned around. Without exception they looked harmless, terrified even. These prisoners did not need to be locked up for society's safety. They were here for punishment.

Female offenders tend to commit fraud and other non-violent crimes, but still I was intrigued to find out what crimes had resulted in their imprisonment. You realise as a prison visitor you should refrain from asking someone what the reason is for their imprisonment. I did ask the interpreter, though, about the sort of crimes, in general, they might have committed that resulted in their incarceration. He said a variety of offences, which, like in most countries; revolve around income generating scams to raise money to buy drugs. Female prisoners the world over are twice as likely as male ones to have a drug problem.

As we entered the first prison cell, I was surprised at how large, airy and light it was. Two bunk beds were pushed up against two walls that met at a corner. White cotton makeshift curtains hanged down from the top bunk, softening the metal bedframes and hiding the bottom bunk bed. The prisoners' eyes ferreted across the room and back and forth to each member in our party. Then my guide explained the reason for my presence, on this warm sunny day in a female prison in Iran, of all places. He told them I was from Australia examining the programs Iran was implementing to prevent HIV. He informed them of my workshop for prison doctors, where we discussed treating females who had a heroin problem so they could avoid prison. I knew any mention of heroin and ways to avoid prison would be of interest to those who used drugs.

My student and I had delivered a three-day workshop to Iranian prison doctors. The workshop covered everything from sharing syringes and transmitting HIV to conjugal visits, condoms and homosexual sex. I remember thinking how would these Muslim men, as all participants were male, respond to two western women discussing homosexual sex in prison? Homosexual sex is illegal in Iran. Offenders are hanged. But the participants were all doctors, so I had hoped that they were pragmatic about the repertoire of human sexual behaviour. One key topic was strategies to prevent HIV. In practice it was rather straightforward, but in reality, many issues hindered prevention. Homophobia and a dislike of drug users discouraged prison authorities from providing condoms and other assistance. Even though methadone is a very effective treatment, authorities disliked it because it is a powerful narcotic drug with euphoric qualities. Most prison authorities preferred that inmates went cold turkey even if that approach was a resounding failure. It was unclear whether our proposed HIV prevention actions were going to be embraced or rejected outright.

My guide went on to say 'This week we have been visiting prisons around the country.' I had hoped this went some way to building a rapport between us. I complimented them on their children and was keen to know how long a baby or child could stay with its mother in prison. Elsewhere, mothers can keep their child for several months or maybe a year or two if they're lucky but then the child is taken from its mother. But some children here were much older than that so I was curious about the rules on this issue. Over the next 30 minutes, we chatted about their families and their children, the ones with them and the ones at home.

One baby-faced girl, who was just a teenager—17, 18, maybe 19 years old but no more—said 'I'm happy with most things.' I was surprised at her volunteering this information; as if it was scripted. But then an elderly tired lady said 'Things are fine; these young people complain about anything.' Maybe the elderly lady knew the youngster had a complaint coming as she cut her off. I asked the elderly lady if she had been here long. Details about the length of someone's prison sentence can give an idea of what sort of crime they might have committed. But she threw me when she said 'This time, ten months. Last time, two years and...' her voice trailed off as she waved a dismissive hand indicating that was all she wanted to say. She was a drug user, 50-something-years old. It wasn't just her multiple prison sentences that gave her away; it was also her swollen hands that revealed a history of injecting into her arm for some years, decades even. The adulterants that were added to heroin had damaged her veins, clogging them up and hindering the blood from circulating to her hands. I surmised she no longer injected into her arm's crook but was sticking the needle into her hands and probably into her legs, her groin area, even. Then another one woman piped up and said, 'the food is good and we have access to a doctor but I'm looking forward to getting out so I can return home to see my family.' So mostly they were happy; well, at least in front of our party.

Then my guide wondered if I would care to speak to the women without any staff present. I was astounded by this offer and hastily accepted, in case there had been a mistake, or someone might object and rescind the offer. My interpreter stayed with me while everyone else departed. By now we had accumulated quite an entourage of five curious onlookers who all watched me as they filed out. And there I stood in the middle of a cell for female inmates in Iran. I was so unprepared. I held my breath, not wanting to make a mistake. Ideas swirled around in my mind, while I tried to frame them into questions or comments. I was unsure if I should even ask them anything, chat or invite questions from them. The interpreter picked up on my apprehensiveness and suggested perhaps they could tell me if they had any complaints about the prison. My anxiety grew as it was unclear what I could do about their complaints. Pass them onto the authorities? How had I become some go-between?

Every pair of eyes focused tightly on me. Inmates waited for me to begin. Then a well-groomed woman who had been watching our exchanges asked if I was married. This ice breaker was usually followed by how many children do you have? Rather than do you have any at all? I had to admit I wasn't married, and I had no children. This was met with 'Tsk, Tsk' while she pursed her lips and shook her head. So I asked her if she was married and how many children she had. This line of inquiry seemed an acceptable thread to pursue. Then I broached the topic of how they were faring. This opening meant they could take it up however they pleased. This approach also excused me from leading the conversation. What if some travesty was recounted to me? Was the discussion destined to venture onto topics that should not be shared with a visiting foreigner?

'I'm not getting all my medication,' a frustrated lady in her mid-twenties exclaimed. She looked weary and seriously underweight. Although all wore the same chador, hers was faded and swamped her tiny frame. She seemed quite annoyed about her predicament. Hers was a common complaint among drug users; I guessed they always felt like they were being swindled. Nevertheless, I decided to explore her complaint.

'What sort of medication are you on?' I asked.

She said 'I should get pills to put me to sleep but I don't get enough, I don't sleep at night.'

Another explanation for her insomnia could be due her being dependent on sleeping pills and that she required more pills to induce sleep. Insomnia was a typical problem for many inmates. Prisons were filled with noises of people fighting, screaming, gates shamming shut and PA announcements. And prison wings were full to the brim of damaged, crazy and loud people. Finally, one young woman said 'I want to get off heroin but I can't do it. If someone helped me outside, I wouldn't be here now.' She was right. If drug users received treatment in the community, they were less likely to end up in jail.

More women came forward, with more complaints. I just sighed and looked at the interpreter. He set about gathering a pen and notepaper to record their issues and promised to raise them with the prison director. I felt compelled to participate. I was unable to extricate myself from this impromptu roundtable of complaints about the prison, their lives and soon enough husbands. Chairs were brought to us to form a circle where we listened to their complaints, tumbling out one after another.

We duly listed them and promised to inform them what could be done. The complaints were not so serious and seemed to be reasonable. Just then my guide returned to the cell and asked us if we were ready to move on. We bid them farewell and there was much grabbing and holding of hands and hugging. They kept saying *Lotfan* and *Merci*, please and thank you in that order, over and over again.

As we moved along a sparse white corridor, we passed more cells on both sides. The parallel rows of florescent lights on the ceiling without any metal cage covering them called out to be smashed. The several chandeliers each with a dozen glass candles hanged from the ceiling, tempting an angry inmate to destroy them. Next, we came upon a large room filled with plants. I quickly surmised it was a waiting room for the doctor and a busy one at that. Prison-based doctors were either very dedicated or worked there because they couldn't work anywhere else.

The waiting room was spotless and tidy. We stopped at the doctor's surgery and I briefly wondered if this was where I should offload all the complaints I had gathered down the corridor. But no opportunity presented itself. Next, we went to the vocation rooms where there were plenty of work opportunities and activities. A huge loom sat in the corner with two inmates twisting their fingers around the warp threads. The steps of a mosque had begun to materialise at the bottom of the weaving. In another corner several girls who were making hair pins giggled when I approached them. '*Salam*,' I said, and they just giggled some more. Why these girls were incarcerated in an adult prison was a mystery. My enthusiastic guide motioned it was time to move on as a female worker gave me an assortment of their handicrafts, which were very appealing. One item which stood out was a beaded sheaf for a pen, which sounds simple but was rather beautiful.

As we continued on our excursion through the prison, we approached the main entrance. A cluster of prison entrants was milling around the reception room. All were adorned in the same black chador. I motioned that I was curious to enter, and the guide obliged me. Twenty-five to 30 very restless women darted about, whispering to each other. Some may have been withdrawing from drugs and others were maybe just plain nervous. Perhaps some still carried drugs on their person, desperate to dump them. A video about HIV was playing on the screen high up in the corner but no one was watching. It appeared they were newcomers, about to undergo the reception process. For a newcomer to prison, this procedure can be daunting. It often involved a medical assessment and furnishing personal details about one's sex life and drug-taking history.

The guide was summonsing us to follow. Our sojourn had taken several hours and was unscheduled. At the end of corridor, we were ushered into a large meeting room filled with an enormous wooden boardroom table. Here we were joined by a senior staffer who was keen to listen to my impressions of the establishment. The staffer seemed to have some authority, but I missed hearing what exactly was her position

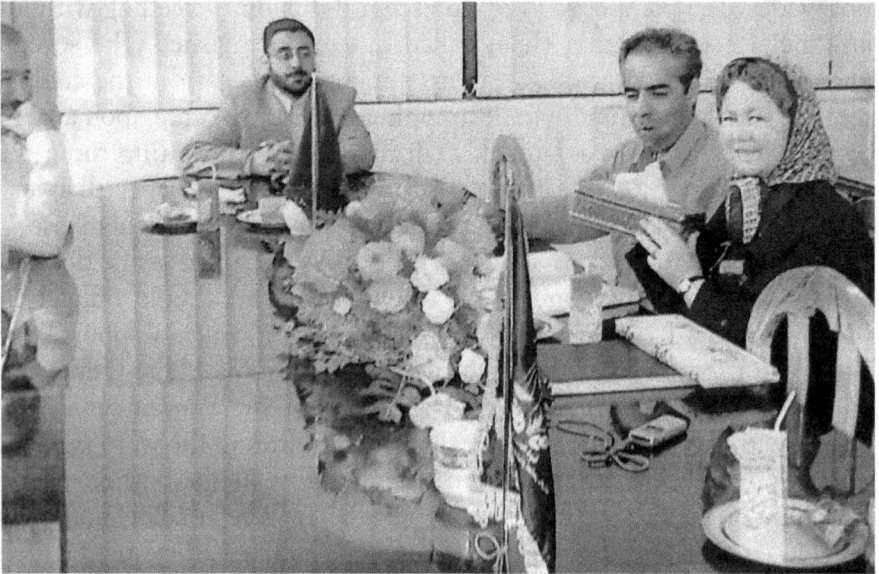

The author meets with prison officials after visiting Evin prison

Sitting around one end of the table, we smiled and introduced ourselves. At the far end of the table was a collection of pint-size Iranian flags on stands, which presumably were brought out for important meetings. First, tea was served with fruit and biscuits. I had already sipped my way through four cups of tea in the prison. 'What is your impression of our prison?' the staffer asked me directly. I had been truly impressed with the prison; even the food I had eaten for lunch was delicious but simple comprising rice, vegetables and large flat bread made by the inmates. She could sense a reservation or two and pushed on again, directly asking me if there were any other issues. As our conversation was being translated, there was a slight pause while each question and answer ping ponged back and forth between us via the interpreter. I complimented her tireless dedicated workers and the HIV education blaring out of the telly at the newcomers. Once more she asked, prompting me to think now might be the moment to pass on those weighty complaints. A glance to my companions for their views was futile. Tentatively, I began to broach the subject and hinted that several women had made some rumblings. A more intent look at my guide and interpreter drew them into the discussion. I nodded at them for confirmation, also pleading for their support. They acquiesced. I casually mentioned that one woman thought she had received only some of her due medication. The staffer identified her immediately by name. The guide confirmed the complainant was her. Apparently, Fatima made this complaint often. A second complainant was concerned with another inmate who most likely had a mental health issue as she lacked basic social skills. She was fighting and stealing from, and arguing with, anyone within her reach. The complainant wanted her belongings returned.

Realising that they did not require me to raise their complaints was a welcomed relief. Their complaints were known. Now I felt able to tackle another issue. Whether there were any plans to provide methadone therapy to them. Our tour of the men's prisons focused on that. But before my question was translated the staffer butted in that this was scheduled to happen in good time. Obviously, this was a prickly point. The guide chimed in confirming how treatment aided them to avoid prison, a well-known fact from thousands of studies in our field. As the meeting came to a close, gifts were presented and we posed for photos. I was glad to be leaving prison on that stifling hot September day in 2003.

*

As we stepped out into the beating sun after leaving Evin Prison, my guide and I sought out another cup of tea, in the city this time. My guide, who had by this time collected his daughter, escorted me down alleyway after alleyway to our destination—an ancient teahouse with gigantic rugs on the floor and the walls. Busy young waiters floated around serving patrons. A waiter came over and beckoned us to follow him towards the back of the teahouse, which was enchantingly cloaked in history. Groups of men smoked hookah pipes, laughing amongst themselves and waving at us. Through the smoky atmosphere, the vaulted ceiling sat miles away, like a crypt. My guide insisted I try the hookah pipe, ignoring my resistance. The intense dose of tobacco made me dizzy and nauseous and fixed me to the rug.

Our attention turned to our tour around his fascinating country; the men in prison, and to the women in Evin Prison. Would he make sure the complaints were addressed? I quizzed him. Yes, of course, he placated me and informed me that the female sex was always complaining, and he just laughed. During our jaunt, we had become firm friends. Despite the haze in my head, it was in that Tehran teashop that the seeds of an idea were sown. Though no clear plan existed yet, the idea of a service for Iranian females was born as we sat cross-legged on musty ruby red rugs.

We reminisced about our incredible journey to eight prisons in the last ten days. It was a privilege to gain an insight into a country's misgivings and its compassion. At one institution, I met murderers on death row and without warning. In that particular prison we entered a large room with huge rugs covering the floor. One doctor wondered if I was afraid. I was unsure why he was checking and then proceeded to inform me that all these men, the 15 or so men milling around us, were on death row and had nothing to lose. Thoughts raced through my mind as I repeated the phrase 'nothing to lose.' Um, did he mean if they attacked us or killed us? I imagined few westerners dropped by their vocational room. Momentarily I considered my safety but realised I had to trust him. Then the reason for the presence of an extra guard was apparent now. He had tailed us since we entered this room and was shadowing me in particular. I felt I owed him a grateful smile. Apparently, many death row inmates weren't executed but were pardoned. The family of their victim has the right to kill them by kicking the stool from under them while they were strung up. Or they can pardon the offender. Many were pardoned; revenge was not what people wanted as it failed to heal the family's hurt. Families, however, wanted justice, which meant the offender would have to serve a considerable amount of prison time.

One stop was a prison in the South of Iran which is surrounded by blue grey mountains. Our guide insisted we alight from our car outside the prison's perimeter and walk in through the prison gate. As the gate rolled back into the wall, we were confronted by a strange pile of sandbags that were right in the centre of the prison yard. It was an art installation apparently, a replica of a bunker from the Iran-Iraq war. To enter the bunker, one had to crouch down to an awkward position and inch in. Once inside and when our eyes had adjusted to the dim light, there was a silhouette of an Iranian soldier, knelt down in prayer. On his left maps were scattered on the dirt floor, and to his right was a wooden bookstand holding a book, the Koran, presumably. Rays of light seeped through the gaps between the sandbags illuminating the dusty air giving an eerie feeling. When Iran was invaded by Iraq in 1980, my guide had served in the medical camps treating the injured. He shook his head and pursed his lips. The war dragged on for eight years, over half a million lives were lost and many more were maimed. The war was also notorious for Saddam Hussein's use of chemical warfare. I left the bunker thinking how horrible that war must have been.

We were escorted around the prison yard and came across a bunch of guys playing basketball. Our guide joined in the game. One of the players was HIV positive and was allowed to freely associate with his fellow inmates. Back then many countries segregated HIV positive inmates. Before we left an aid asked us to pose for photos. As we exited the prison, I was presented with framed photographs of my time inside. The frames were made in the marquetry style, which featured an inlay of a golden pattern of stars in a wooden frame.

As the time came to leave prison for the day, I began to wonder where our hotel was. But to my amazement we were to spend the night in prison, in the staff quarters. This trip had just begun and already it was surreal. How often was a visit to prison followed by an overnight stay inside? Of all my trips to numerous prisons over many years, I had never slept inside one. It was unnerving but I had no other choice.

I was a little apprehensive to be in a room by myself. Staff kept checking on me, but I was not game to venture out of my little haven. Instead, I stared out at the beautiful, blue mountains. The terrain was very jagged, like torn paper with green and blue watercolours dabbed across it. Strange thoughts started to occupy me; no one knew where I was, apart from my travelling companions. What if there was a prison riot? I did not sleep well that night.

*

Our chat at the teahouse was interrupted by a busy waiter serving plates of intriguing dishes. Before us he laid out *piyaz torshi*, pickled onions, *chelow kabab*, rice and roasted meat and some Nan bread to have with a bowl of *ash-e anār*, a soup made with pomegranates. Our attention turned to our visit to the prison in Mashhad, with both of us breaking into laughter. As soon as we arrived at the airport we headed straight to prison. The guide summoned a guard to bring an inmate to us. I had no idea what was about to transpire. The inmate was ordered upstairs to an office. We followed in single file and sat by several desks, waiting. Soon it became apparent that this fellow was some sort of computer whizz who had designed a computerised medical records system for the prison. Presumably the inmate was convicted of a white-collar crime. The interpreter stood up in protest. He brought a new slant on the moment by pleading that tomorrow was a more appropriate time, instead of 2 am. Of course, he was correct, but I was astounded that no one else, not even me, had registered how strange this scenario was. So off we trundled to our hotel and came back the next day, at a more reasonable hour, when it was daylight and after breakfast.

The next day we called in on a painting class for inmates. Most were quite skilled at painting and some had painted murals on the prison walls. Most of the murals depicted how illicit drugs can kill you and turn you against your family. Other classes on offer were motor mechanics, architecture and literacy. Further along we came across some building works being carried out by inmates. Several guys walked around with all manner of tools, which seemed an enormous amount of trust to be placed in the hands of criminals. One fellow passed me with a plane that is used to smooth cement. Another had a hammer! It was clear both workers could cause serious injury with their tools, but they didn't and weren't about to.

This trip had become some distorted adventure that was perplexing to comprehend. Our guide was hurrying us along to another surprize, no doubt. This time it was a row of prison cells without doors; huge gaps stood where the doors should be. Inmates could walk in and out at their leisure. About 12 to 15 men resided in each one. He wondered if I cared to peek inside and I nodded and smiled, nervously. As I moved towards the cell, he first needed to ask the residents for their permission. After a brief exchange in Farsi, we were invited into their cell. Oddly they wore regular street clothes and rather smart ones. One fellow had a pencil-thin moustache, a burgundy polar neck jumper, cream linen trousers and leather shoes that laced up slightly off centre. He was very near to me, a little too close, as close as two dancers might be. His dark eyes looked directly into mine then his face broke into a grin. As I glanced round the cell, all eyes were on me, a western Anglo woman just inside the door of their cell. They questioned my colleagues as to my reason for

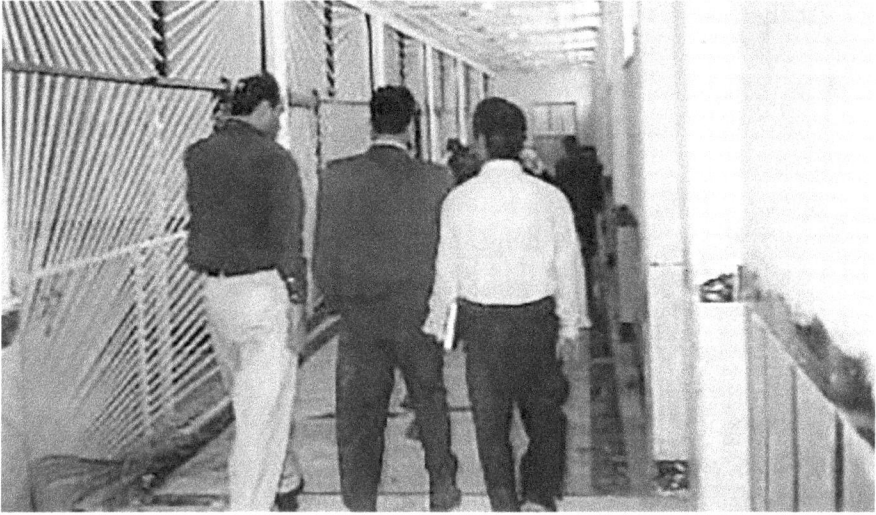

Sunray-shaped bars on prison cells

being there, I surmised by their gesturing. Some reason was provided which met with their approval. Their demeanour was of impeccable politeness, offering me a seat on one of the bunk beds, which my guide declined on my behalf. As we departed their cell, the guide pointed out the shape of the bars on the walls of the cells. They were fashioned to resemble the rays of sunshine. I inquired if they ever absconded, but no reply was given.

Questions were asked of me as we walked along the corridor. Did we in the West lock inmates in their cells, and wasn't that unkind. Another titillating feature awaited us as we ventured further into the prison complex. After negotiating several short corridors, we came upon a bedroom. The décor was rather dated, a red satin bedspread on a wrought iron bed framed by a huge bedhead. A small table to one side held condoms and lubricants with a bin tucked underneath. It was a private meeting room, a sacred room for inmates to have a conjugal visit with their spouse. Apparently, no matter how they behaved, inmates were entitled to these visits. This adventure was so challenging to comprehend. Few countries offer this fringe benefit for those detained by society. However, it was easy to imagine how such a service kept a family together, and warded off sexual frustration.

*

At the teahouse and by our third cup of tea we wrestled with some unresolved issues. Where were the gaps in Iran's response to HIV? Were they in their prison system? My guide believed more services for female prisoners was the answer. I argued for their release or better still not being locked up. This required changes to the law, which could take an eon, even in Iran. Also, a legal expert would have to be recruited into our mission and adopt this challenge as it sat outside our areas of expertise. Every suggestion was rebuffed by the other. After some lively debate we wondered if it was females in prison who had the greatest unmet need. But what should we do next? We sat in silence sipping our sweet tea. My trip around Iran had indicated that anything could be achieved in Iran, even the unimaginable. Finally, we agreed it was females in the community who needed the most help, to stay out of prison, and so it was decided that we should set about establishing a centre for female drug users. As we departed from the teahouse, I felt elated and optimistic, but also stumped as to what our next move would entail.

I remembered our visit to Isfahan, which is situated in the middle of the country. It has a wonderful reputation for its craftsmanship. I remembered the stunning *Khaju* Bridge with its lovely lights illuminating 13 arches over the *Zayandeh* River. A few foreign tourists were milling around the markets, and I was amused by how much they stood out. One lady was wearing her hejab like a skullcap with the material rolled up around the edge. Only then did I realise that I was probably also standing out in my unorthodox hejab. A little further along at a haberdashery stall, I bought a brightly coloured hand printed calico bedspread. A tired old large man was sitting behind a desk printing the pattern onto cloth in the shop. The poor old fellow had a stamp tied to his hand and he just kept pounding the ink pad and then the cloth making a pattern of flowers and vines. It was a gorgeous pattern, though I'm sure his wrist had suffered permanent damage from all that stamping. We wandered through the bazaar looking at the different stalls.

While we flew to Isfahan, our onward passage was by car. Sanctions had impacted on aviation safety, with new parts for planes being unavailable. While my guide apologized for this change in our mode of transport, I was pleasantly surprised to be driven through the countryside. I was struck by how mountainous it was. Steep rough cliffs surrounded us.

I had begged my guide to show me something other than prisons in his stunning country. He took me to see Persepolis, the capital of the Persian Empire. Persepolis sits in the South West corner of Iran. It was built in about 500 BC and comprised royal palaces, halls and a treasury where gold and silver were stored. I sat in the shade and did some sketching. Soon I was surrounded by kids sneaking a peek at my sketch pad to judge whether my drawing resembled the object being drawn. A young boy sidled up to me and obviously wanted to draw, too. I tore off a page and handed it to him. Then I positioned my pastels within his reach. He smelt of homelessness, his hair was matted, and he had not bathed for some time. He was a street kid who begged at the ruins. My attention returned to my sketch of the two pillars, which stood on top of a marble staircase. The boy clutched a pastel, began to draw, kept drawing, and did not stop. His drawing did not resemble anything in front of him but rather something inside him. He was depicting a story, and at a frenzied pace, but used only one colour; black. A green pastel stick was pushed next to his paper, but he was so absorbed he failed to notice. Then, all of a sudden, he stopped and smiled and motioned that he wanted to take his drawing with him. I nodded and off he skipped with his drawing.

Afterwards we drove around the town, checking out some touristy sites. Then it was back to work. My guide showed me where he had facilitated perhaps the first group for drug users in his country and then we called on an old client of his. The guy had struggled through life; he appeared old and haggard and malnourished. At his home, we were ushered into a large simple room with a huge wall hanging of a forest scene at the opposite end. Rugs and large cushions covered the floor. His wife seemed happy enough considering she had lived with a chronic drug user for some 30 years. Later, I discovered he was an opium smoker. It was fascinating to be invited into these folks' home. Although resources were tight in this household, they were incredibly hospitable, offering food and refreshments and the best cushion in the house. The room had practically no furniture in it. And everyone seemed content to sit on the floor on a rug. Being unaccustomed to sitting on the floor for long periods, I curled up in a corner on two large cushions and fell asleep. Later I was worried that I was probably snoring and, when I quizzed my guide, he commented that I might have purred, just a little.

Next on our whistle stop tour of Iran was Shiraz, a stunning city and home of the famous poet, Hafez. On a bright sunny day, we drove to an oasis, the Musalla Gardens on the banks of the Rukn-Abad River. The spectacular Gardens were in full bloom, yet surrounded by dusty plains. Once inside the walls, which were trimmed with aqua blue ceramic tiles with inlays, I spotted Hafez's tomb. It was a large open rotunda sitting high on five circular steps. Around the edge of the top step, eight pillars supported a domed-shape roof. At night, the intricate patterned ceiling was illuminated showing blues, reds and purples that reflected back down on the tomb. Inside the rotunda was a marble tombstone inscribed with several of the poet's verses. The inmates at the local prison gave me a wooden replica of his tomb that they had made in their woodwork class.

Then Yazd was on the agenda; in the South East, this time to visit a young offenders' institution. Yazd was the centre of Zoroastrian culture with about half a million inhabitants. It had a reputation for its fine silk rugs and delicious sweets. I couldn't remember agreeing to all these site visits, or even knowing about them. All this travelling had become tiresome and I was homesick. But I had to push on as this opportunity was unique. The institution was rather small and compact. The youths looked like regular kids. But these young teens were embarking on a passage to become adults, and whether that included a stint in an adult prison no one knew. They seemed keen to convince us they had plans to head back to school and away from trouble. We could have chosen to focus our efforts on the young offenders, but instead females were to be our focus.

On our way back to Tehran, we drove through very sparse countryside so I loosened my hejab, allowing it to slip down around the nape of my neck. It was dark and I thought they won't notice or if they did, surely, they wouldn't fuss about it now. I began to think what if these guys wanted to do away with me? I could go missing quite easily out here. Then I reminded myself they were doctors, bound by the Hippocratic Oath. So I reclined in my seat and dozed off sans hejab.

I couldn't believe the difficulties I had faced to visit Iran, given the amazing nature of this trip. When my guide had invited me to visit Iran in 2003, I had to make a request at my research centre for permission to visit Iran. Although I had funds specifically for this purpose, I still needed my boss' approval. My boss was less than enthusiastic about this trip. I had planned to take two colleagues with me, but he put a stop to that. I managed to persuade him to allow my PhD student, Carolyn, to accompany me. He was lukewarm on these foreign projects. He once told me that my Program of International Research and Training was not about international work at all, in spite of the name. I was determined not to let this lack of support deter me. Then our visa applications had been left languishing on someone's desk at the Iranian embassy in Canberra for about six months. Once we realised that we needed a sponsor, it was possible to obtain a visa. We just didn't know the process. On the application form you had to sign that you would observe all the laws and regulations applicable to foreign nationals, including the dress code for women.

After our trip around the country, we had a free day. My PhD student was eager to track down a street named after the Irish hunger striker Bobby Sands, who died in a Northern Irish prison in 1981. The British Embassy sat on Winston Churchill Street in Tehran. In a show of solidarity, the Iranians renamed the road Bobby Sands Street. The British Embassy responded by shifting their front entrance to a side street, to avoid using a street named after the hunger striker.

I was due to depart Iran in the next few days but not before a final debriefing meeting at the United Nations' Head Office. Although the UN had not been involved in my visit, they were keen to meet me and hear my impressions of Iran's response to HIV. The meeting had been arranged rather hastily, so I hadn't had much time to prepare. My fellow travelling companions were invited as well. I wondered if the ideas we explored at the teahouse the previous day would feature at the meeting. During this first trip to Iran, I had been escorted everywhere, but now I was making my own way in a taxi. The taxi took me through some parts of Tehran where I hadn't previously travelled. I had the address written down and a map so I was content to daydream as we weaved through the streets and traffic of North Tehran. We passed a synagogue, one of the 35 in Iran, which the taxi driver went to some lengths to point out to me. Then we passed a large mosque, again he was poking the air for me to see. Hundreds of shoes lined the entrance waiting for their owners to collect them. It was time for the midday prayers, or *Zuhr*, which began after the sun has crossed the zenith point.

The taxi pulled into the UN driveway crunching gravel as it neared a wide, low white building. As we approached, I saw the walls were extremely thick, with guards posted at the gate. I showed my passport and presented an invitation letter from the person I was to meet.

Although I had yet to meet the UN lady, I had heard about her and knew she held progressive views. She looked very cosmopolitan. I kept looking at her hejab and thinking why doesn't mine look like hers? She had it draped over her head and shoulders and across her chest. And it sat so elegantly in place. It had a tapestry type print on it. I felt like I was wearing a nylon football scarf from a losing team. She ushered me into her office and then proceeded to remove her hejab. Women were required to wear the veil in the early 1900s, but not from 1936 to 1979 and then again after the 1979 Revolution. Whether they should cover their hair with a veil was debated often. Relieved, I shed my hejab, too. I had been experimenting with various styles and couldn't seem to find a comfortable way of wearing it. In one style I tried, I saw my grandmother looking at me in the mirror. We both smoked cigarettes. I choked. These Iranian cigarettes, like many in the developing world, were always strong to very strong, and they stank. Soon her other guests arrived, and we were shepherded into a meeting room and offered more tea, biscuits and fruit.

Introductions gave way to polite conservations, which carried on for some time. The UN had invited a range of colleagues who worked in the HIV field and were keen to hear about Australian programs. It was well known that Australia had averted an epidemic of HIV, even in Iran. It must have been about our second cup of tea that the guy, who I assumed was the most devout Muslim in the room, demanded that I advise them what they should do to stop AIDS. He wore the obligatory beard and had previously chastised me for having a few curls poke out of my hejab. He became serious declaring that condoms were available in prisons, for when wives visit… but then he stopped that line of conversation as if he didn't want to acknowledge homosexual sex occurred in prison. Conjugal visits almost certainly reduced homosexual sex. Islam, as I had come to appreciate, was a very compassionate religion and a case could be made for the lesser of two evils. He implied that homosexual sex was a lesser evil than an AIDS death, so condom provision could be justified. But was the Koran that flexible?

I struggled to comprehend this. Islam may appear rigid to the casual eye, but actually it is an adaptable way of life. In Islam, one is encouraged to lead a healthy, active life with the qualities of kindness, chastity, honesty, mercy, courage, patience and politeness. We skirted around sticky topics. He demanded again that I inform them exactly what to do, and then he would make it sit well with the Koran. I couldn't imagine how certain programs could ever be palatable to most religions, let alone Islam. Activities had to cater for prostitutes, transsexuals and perhaps, most poignantly, females with a drug problem. I caught my guide's eye and he encouraged me to continue, so the areas I thought worthy of the most attention were listed. How he could repackage it into something acceptable to followers of Islam was beyond me. I was in disbelief.

As the meeting continued, the topic moved to the judiciary and how judges could play a role in reducing harms by diverting drug users from prison to treatment. I outlined the role these key people played in Australia. They seemed interested so I suggested the judiciary visit Australia to inspect our drug courts. I urged them to consider who they sent to prison, those who looked and probably were harmless. A three-pronged approach was needed for women. The first group was to be the women already imprisoned, the second group was those about to be discharged from prison and the third group was the women in the community who were to be prevented from another stint in prison. Pragmatism reigned in Iran. Who knew that when you ventured to some far away country you would be astounded by what people were trying to do to prevent HIV from spreading and all in the name of Allah? *Inshallah.*

As our meeting came to an end, I presented the UN lady with a book on Australia with stunning photos of our beaches and rainforests. She seemed a little embarrassed as she handed over a small coarse rug to me as a parting gift. The rug was about a metre square; half was turquoise and half was a sandy colour. Depicted diagonally across the middle of the rug was an enormous opium pipe with a tiny woman lying on her back on it, skewered by a needle. Three figures stood by watching in one corner, a woman in a brown chador and two children. In another corner was the UN logo comprising a world map with the initials UNDCP, the United Nations Drug Control Program, albeit upside down. Today the rug sits in the centre of my study. Judging by the theme of the design, I inquired as to who had made it. Apparently, there was a competition for students to design patterns for rugs that were woven by female inmates. Strangely, it was the weavers of this rug—female drug users—who were to become the focus of my research for the next decade.

As my first trip came to an end, I spent my last night with my guide. My plane left very late in the night and I was exhausted. I had

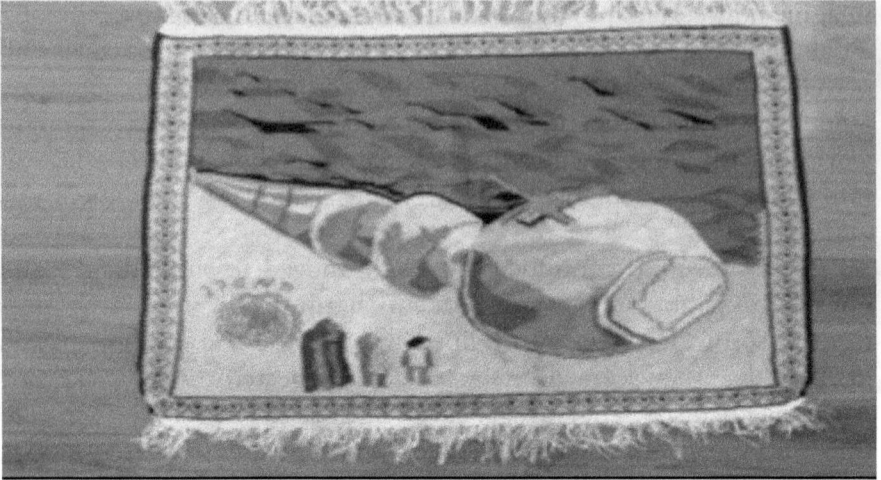

A rug made by female inmates that was a gift from the UN lady

excess luggage and had to negotiate the excess baggage system. I had accumulated so much stuff, including the mandatory Persian rug, a pale green silk one with intricate patterns on it. My guide gave me a tan vinyl suitcase to carry all my presents home. I had been presented with many gifts from the prisoners; a wood carving depicting two men from a wall of the ruins in Persepolis, another present was a fine wooden mosaic of a woman holding a jug on her shoulder standing over a man near a tree. The old man looked like he might be a poet. On the back they had written 'dedicated to Professor Kate Dolan by Central Prison of Isfahan, Iran *Hayat Al-Ghaib* Chief of Central Prison 3/6/82.' That was 1382. I also received stone statues of winged horses from Persepolis and a blue glass decanter and glasses set. Perhaps the most wonderful present was a wooden model of Hafez's tomb. It seemed to be an exact replica and the prison director had written a lovely message to me on its base.

The airport system for paying for excess baggage was difficult to grasp as none of the women at the counters spoke English and I hadn't mastered Farsi. A fellow passenger pointed upstairs so up I went only to be sent back down to drag my three suitcases up. The cases needed to be weighed upstairs to determine the duty to be paid. I struggled to move my bags upstairs one at a time and downstairs again, one at a time but finally managed to check in and board my plane.

Chapter 2. Back to Sydney

After returning to Sydney from my first trip to Iran, I told Margaret, my partner, about the trip and the women in prison in particular. We had stayed up all night dissecting the trip; she was worried as she hadn't heard from me at all while I was in Iran. She said 'Well, you should do something for the women in prison; what can you do for them?' And it was the last thing she ever said to me.

The next day I was woken by laboured breathing and rushed into the lounge room to find Margaret unconscious and struggling to breathe. She had thrown her glasses across the room. I couldn't rouse her, so I called an ambulance. Immediately I put her on the floor and commenced mouth to mouth resuscitation and chest compressions. I didn't think to feel for a pulse but soon the ambulance workers arrived and took over. They cut her clothes off and placed paddles on her chest to start her heart beating. As soon as it started, they said let's get her to hospital. I was worried but I thought that with time a full recovery was to be expected. At the hospital she was admitted to the emergency department and, when I was prevented from any contact for several hours, I began to realise the seriousness of the situation.

I was stuck with a social worker who was just hopeless. I rang a friend, Jen, and she came and sat with me and we just waited; we had to call all of Margaret's sisters, five in total. And the sister who was the closest to her flew down from Brisbane immediately. Her sisters were asking Jen whether they should come down, but Jen replied that it was their decision, she could just update them what was happening here. I spent the night at the hospital but didn't get any sleep. So I decided I should return home each night to sleep as I had to make decisions about her treatment. Two friends turned up with six bottles of beer to visit her in intensive care. I was very disappointed that they hadn't realised the seriousness of the situation. I told them to take the beer away, then one came back with some sleeping pills for me; I guess they just didn't know how to help. The nurse started saying it been 48 hours now and I quickly corrected him that it was just 24 hours, so whatever assessment you are making is wrong if it's based on time. I actually felt in control of the situation insofar as I was able to discuss things with the doctor and nurses and the five sisters and remain calm and be the contact person for staff, friends and family alike. The next day wasn't much better; by this time our doctor friends had started to come by to see how she was. She was in an induced coma as she had been fitting. I found out more details; she had several heart attacks in the emergency department. Each one had caused more damage to her heart and to her brain.

Alex, who had been a supervisor to both of us when we did our PhDs, visited her in hospital and then left to catch a plane. But the plane had a mechanical fault, a flat battery, and so he returned. I couldn't believe it. I thought if I had the chance to evade this situation I surely would. I had no experience of death, of dying, of hospitals or seriously ill people. Throughout the day her sisters began arriving one by one to hold a vigil by her bedside. The diagnosis of Margaret became progressively worse. The doctor expected improvement; she should find the tubes annoying but I was arguing she was sedated so how can she object to the tube down her throat? Then another doctor said she isn't breathing on her own and I knew she was and told him. He went and checked the medical notes and he came back and agreed. The next day she had an MRI scan and our worse fears were realised. She had grade 4 damage to her brain, meaning complete incapacitation. A grade 3 rating might have given someone a chance with rehabilitation, but grade 4 was considered beyond help. It didn't take long for her family to discuss this. And I led the discussion that it was better to let her go in peace than to hang on to her. One sister was confused about the diagnosis, but once it was explained again to her, she agreed.

I had spent some time listening to Margaret talk about her brother who had been kept on life support for years after a bike accident. Margaret had made her views on this issue very clear over the years. That he should not be resuscitated and had this marked on his chart. We were told she had no chance of recovery and, as she was in a Catholic hospital, euthanasia was not an option. So Margaret was now in a vegetative state and possibly in some pain. Although she had been breathing on her own, she was on a breathing tube. It was unknown what response was likely if, and when, we decided to take her off life support.

I instructed Greg, Margaret's supervisor to summons the doctor so I could inform him of our decision. There should be no delay. We had her sisters here so we should do it now. I was watching this tragedy unfold like I was somehow detached from my body.

We called the priest, Father Laurie, who had visited her to perform the last rites and to offer some comfort to us. Then the breathing tube was removed, and we waited. As she struggled for breath, I found it unbearable to sit by her bedside in intensive care. I went home with tears streaming down my face. After a little while I got the call at 10 pm—she had passed away. We sat at our dining room table, the one I had shared daily with Margaret, and opened a bottle of Château Margot from France that I had bought for her on an earlier trip. All her sisters stayed that night at our place, for the first time.

Tuesday, we proceeded to make funeral plans, visiting the undertaker to decide on the type of coffin, the format for the service and where she was to be buried. Should the plot be a double one where I might be buried too? We were able to view the body. My mum had come up and came to the viewing, though she didn't view the body. I had written a heartfelt letter to Margaret, telling her what had happened, how she had suffered several heart attacks, how her brain had been damaged, beyond repair. And that I loved her. I placed a few personal items in her casket, her favourite pastels, some police crime scene tape that had been a joke between us and my letter. She would be buried in a shroud.

I had to purchase some new clothes for the funeral. I had a black pillbox hat made with a small veil covering my eyes. I bought waterproof mascara. I expected to cry. I wore sunglasses and a dress Margaret had made me, a deep purple satin dress. Some nights we used to venture out dressed up as Jackie O and Doris Day to dance in nightclubs. She would wear a pillbox hat and me a blonde wig.

The funeral was held on Friday at the Prince Henry Hospital Chapel on the rugged coast at Little Bay. The Chapel was a small A-frame building with a long white wooden cross on the roof at the far end. The Chapel's entire back wall was a massive stained-glass window overlooking the ocean, which infused the room with a kaleidoscope of soft colour. It was positioned in the grounds of a golf course that we had played on a few times. Our dear friend, Jackie, sang "Secret Love" and "Crazy" at the funeral. Greg gave a heart moving eulogy and struggled to contain his composure. One sister sobbed as she read from *The Prophet* by Kahlil Gibran. My brother delivered the Gospel according to Matthew. "Whatsoever you do for the least of them, you do for me" (Matthew 25:40). It was such a fitting tribute to Margaret. Father Laurie gave the Homily and spoke as if he knew her. He mentioned that she liked a drink and that she was truly loved. A montage of her life was shown through slides projected onto a screen. An early photo of Margaret in her nurse's hat, a heavily starched cornette, broke the tension in the Chapel with everyone laughing out loud.

The bagpiper started playing "Amazing Grace" as the coffin was taken out of the Chapel and placed in the hearse. The cortege proceeded to the burial site in the Eastern Suburbs Memorial Park. I stood looking up to the sky while her coffin was lowered into the grave. I felt so alone. The funeral party moved on to the wake at another golf course, St Michael's. Here all her friends and family celebrated her memory and expressed their astonishment at how young she was to die. She was fit and full of life just several days ago and now we were attending her wake. After the wake several friends and I visited Oxford Street, and then I met some others at my home. We sat at the table in silence. It was too hard to comprehend.

Some months later the tombstone had to be designed, so I took Jen with me. I had not cried at all at the funeral but now I could not stop. I had to decide on the wording, the type of stone and whether to include a photo of her. These decisions were beyond me. She died intestate. We had just purchased the next door flat and converted the two flats into a large one. I was left with two mortgages, a bank loan for the renovations but just one salary. We had counted on two salaries to repay our loans. It took an eon to negotiate the legal system to be awarded her estate and two of her sisters were not forthcoming in signing the necessary documents.

Chapter 3. How I Came to Work in this Area

My interest in prisoners and prisons began in the mid-eighties—not because I ever had any personal connection, but it was apparent even then that prisons had the potential to become the boiler room of this new epidemic, the HIV epidemic. Alex, my boss, and I discussed the HIV epidemic and how best to respond to it. It had surfaced among junkies in New York, Madrid and Edinburgh. Soon we could expect it on our doorstep in Darlinghurst, a gritty inner-city drug hub suburb of Sydney.

It was 1985 and we were founding members of two groups, one for sex workers, the Australian Prostitutes' Collective and one for drug users, the Australian Drug Information Collective. Collectives were a viable way to mobilise a group around a common goal but often became inefficient after a while. Our monthly meetings had a sizeable overlap of the two groups, Pam, Carol, Julie, Alan, John, Alex, Robyn and me. Debate dominated our meetings for months. When should we break the law and hand out syringes to drug addicts? A HIV screen of patients at Alex's Rankin Court methadone program and four other units detected one person, John, who was HIV positive, the index case. He was from San Francisco so maybe he picked up HIV there? That possibility had to be ruled out. It was Pam's job to trace his sexual and needle contacts. Of the six contacts traced and screened, four tested HIV positive and all were fellow injectors. His long-term girlfriend remained HIV negative as did another needle contact. But of the four HIV positives traced from him, two had shared directly with him while another two had shared with one of his contacts. This contact tracing exercise provided the first evidence that HIV had spread among Sydney's drug-using population. And, as he had been in Sydney for many years, it was there he became infected.

Alex had written 13 submissions to our Department of Health lobbying them to allow us to open a needle and syringe program, but all were declined or ignored. You had to admire his persistence; most would have given up by then. Realising that permission was unlikely, he decided we had to resort to civil disobedience. One day Alex came to me with AUD20 and declared we were commencing tomorrow, so I had to go and buy some needles and syringes. We had lamented over this for two years. Unbeknownst to me, he had been garnering support at his hospital and with the local police commander. The needle and syringe program opened on 13 November 1986. Nobody came that day, but they rolled up the next day. Alex was interviewed at great length by senior detectives down at the police station, who finally decided not to press charges.

A sign on our office building's front door read FREE STERILE NEEDLES AND SYRINGES; BRING IN YOUR OLD ONES. Inside the door was an upside-down milk crate on which sat a box of 100 1ml insulin syringes. On the other side of the door was bustling Victoria Street, Darlinghurst. Word soon spread. The buzzer rang all day and night. I ran up the stairs to answer the door. Clients were asked to put their used syringes in a large sharps bin before receiving new syringes. The only rule was they had to collect two sets of needles and syringes; that way a syringe might be passed onto another without us ever meeting them. I ran the program and coordinated several volunteers. We relied on donations to purchase equipment. Alex had secured some media in the Sunday paper. A call for donations accompanied a story on our program. A week later we had received a single donation, an AUD20 cheque from my aunt Eileen, who mentioned that the news story sounded like the caper I was involved in.

Clients were asked if they wished to make a donation. One day a lady of the night donated AUD20, the exact price of a box of 100 syringes as she had a good shift at work. However, most clients were unable to make a donation, which indicated that this service had to be free.

Staff at the neighbouring methadone unit was unhappy about our needle and syringe program. Every single day a manager from there tore down my sign advertising free fits. When I complained to Alex, he said just put it back up, but don't use thumb tacks; they are marking the door!

With thousands of bloody used syringes being returned, a stack of sharps bins had begun to accumulate under my desk. And we had not thought through how to dispose of them. I suggested having them tested for HIV antibodies.[1] Over the next year, hundreds of returned and used syringes were tested on three separate occasions, delivering three time points of HIV infection in the syringes. The level of HIV infection at each point exceeded the previous one. Sydney was at the

[1] Wodak et al., 1987.

take-off point of an HIV epidemic among its drug injectors. An urgent meeting was requested with the Health Department to discuss these findings and to encourage them to sanction our program and establish more. But they were slow and overly cautious. Instead, they preferred to trial a pharmacy-based scheme where users had to purchase syringes and return them to buy more, albeit at a slight discount. But with the evidence that HIV was here and spreading they had to act. Our needle and syringe program was the third such program in the world. A Dutch drug user group had opened one in response to Hepatitis B in the mid-1980s and Kaleidoscope, a drug agency, began the first UK needle and syringe in 1986. So not only was our project controversial, but the territory was unknown. Some believed dolling out free syringes was likely to encourage the uptake of injecting. One decade later strong evidence had emerged to the contrary.

Officially my work was counseling and advising drug and alcohol users and their family over the telephone, but I was ensconced in our other work—the prostitutes' collective and the drug users' collective. Only one group was to be funded, so we pursued funding for the sex workers first. Newspaper headlines bemoaned the thought that HOOKERS GOT A CUP OF TEA AND A CHAT as if providing a service for sex workers was outrageous. This was an exciting time for me personally as I lived on a boat, no ordinary boat, but an ex-Manly ferry. These ships travelled between Manly in Sydney's North to the city centre, transporting 8,500 passengers at a time. The *Baragoola* was over 200 feet long and moored in the middle of Rozelle Bay, a graveyard bay in Sydney Harbour. I rowed or motored a small boat from the ferry to reach the land every day. When the ferry was sold, I was sad to be moving on.

And soon enough I was lured overseas, to London to evaluate their needle and syringe programs. Gerry Stimson had rung Alex and asked if he knew of anyone who could evaluate the pilot needle and syringe programs in the UK. So off I went, supposedly for two years but staying for six. It was an interesting way to see England and Scotland, visiting the hot spots for drug use and HIV.

Anecdotally, prisons kept popping up as one of the main causes why people were sharing syringes. One day at work I insisted on adding an option to a question in the survey inquiring if anyone had shared a syringe *because* they were in prison. We were prevented from asking interviewees any questions directly about their prison experiences as that was the domain of the Home Office, which outranked the Health

Department. So I secured funding to investigate the prevalence of HIV and the level of risk behaviours by studying ex-prisoners. In this investigation, the level of HIV infection among ex-prisoners would reflect what it was in prison if they were recruited and tested very soon after being release from prison. Our results were in sharp contrast with the Home Office's figures, as ours were ten times higher than theirs. This obviously annoyed the Home Office's HIV expert, Len Curran, a softly spoken Irish man. He would argue that prison is a public place and therefore condoms cannot be provided as its illegal to have sex in a public place. It was disappointing as Len was an out gay man, but he was unable to argue with the establishment.

When I presented the results of this study at the International Conference on AIDS in 1991, Len Curran was the chairperson of my session. He knew the content of my presentation from the abstract book. He then proceeded to introduce himself for the entire time allocated for my presentation. At the end of the session, he declared we were out of time and the session was closed. If anyone wanted to stay back, they could chat to me. He prevented me from delivering my presentation, one that I had practiced for weeks. Nevertheless, our results were published in the *British Medical Journal*[2] and even rated a mention in *Hansard,* the House of Lord's record of debate. That mention declared if only half of what we found was true, the situation was indeed grave.

Tired of being frustrated by the Home Office's resistance to research, I left England and headed home. Once back in Australia, I replicated my UK ex-prisoner study as part of my PhD. I completed another three studies on prisoners and HIV. Of the 498 prisoners I studied, interviewed and met over the years, some died and many caught Hepatitis C, but very few acquired HIV infection. The reason so few injectors became HIV positive was that the needle and syringe program had taken off early in Australia. Only a few inmates became infected with HIV and I had gotten to know them quite well, as I followed them for years. In an outbreak investigation, I had to quite literately trace everyone who had shared a syringe or had sex with my index case, Sam. An index case was the initial patient in an outbreak investigation. I travelled interstate to locate some cases. I traced 13 infected people who had sex or shared a syringe with him. Of the 13 infected contacts; four were definitely infected inside prison and two were definitely infected outside prison. But the location of where the remaining seven were

[2] Turnbull et al., 1992.

infected was indeterminate.[3]

Another dozen or so close contacts who shared a prison cell with Sam were infected within weeks of each other. Their medical files recorded classic seroconversion symptoms, without being identified as such as that condition was still new. The illness usually includes fever, lymphadenopathy, rash, muscle aches, headache, sore throat and diarrhoea. Whether they were infected by Sam was unclear but given that there were fewer than 20 HIV positive inmates in a prison system of 7,000 inmates at that time, then a cluster such as these was highly indicative of an outbreak.[4] We conducted genetic testing of the strain of HIV, like a case in Florida where a dentist infected his patients with his strain of HIV. But the lab reports oscillated from the cases being definitely linked to not being alike at all. This study was incredibly difficult to obtain approval from one ethics committee. The committee seemed to think if we showed someone had infected another then the committee's institution would be held responsible. We had to engage our own lawyer to argue the case with the committee's lawyer.

After a few years Sam had become gravely ill and some prison nurses campaigned for his release. He was granted compassionate release as his life expectancy was severely shortened. I managed to interview him on the outside in Alex's office. While he nodded off, Alex and I chatted about his situation. He had returned to heroin use. At Christmas that year, while watching television with my family, a newsreader reported that Sam was charged with robbery and murder. I remember a relative of mine being rather appalled that I should know such a person. Once I was back at work in the New Year, a prison guard telephoned me and said 'your mate is back inside.' They had my phone number from when I had signed in to enter prison. I debated whether to visit him. I had finished my work with him, but I was curious as to why he had been charged with murder.

We were allowed to meet in prison yard so they could observe us without overhearing our conversation. Sam ranted and raved, waving his hands. When he finished and I walked back to the gate to leave, they teased me that he was chastising me for publishing an article about him becoming infected in prison. But he wasn't: he explained how he accidentally killed someone the previous month. The second time he had murdered someone. This murder happened in a shop he had held

---

[3] Dolan et al., 1994.

[4] Dolan et al., 1994.

up. He told the guy to hand over the money, but instead the guy dropped it, probably in a panic, and to Sam it looked like he was reaching for a gun. And even though he gave several warnings, the shopkeeper did not get up and show his hands were empty. As Sam dipped down to pick up some cash, the gun went off, killing the guy.

His first murder occurred when his friend had made a sexual advance to him and he lost his temper. Once when I interviewed Sam, I requested his prison medical file but when I couldn't locate any serology, I examined it closer and realized that I had been given his father's file by mistake. They had almost identical names. His father was in prison for sexually abusing his children, Sam included.

Whenever I ran a study of prisoners, which was from 1988 to 2019, I always tried to have a serving prisoner sit on the steering committee. Although this added a considerable amount of time as we had to hold the meetings where the prisoner was held and navigate our way through security, it provided a perspective that no one else on the committee could have provided. In Long Bay Prison, we often met in the chapel and Alex chaired the meeting, sitting under a huge crucifix. John, our prison representative had his transsexual girlfriend, Anna, serve tea. Both John and Anna had deliberately infected themselves with HIV in order to be priority cases for methadone treatment.

Previously, my research had focused on HIV, drugs and men as they had made up the bulk of the population of drug users. Although some females featured in a few studies, the bulk of my work had focused on men. So when the opportunity to work with women and to set up a service exclusively for them, I was excited to be righting the balance of my research activities.

Chapter 4. The Drug Scene in Tehran

Iran has a lengthy history of farming and using opium. Its people have smoked opium for centuries. One of the first recorded medicinal uses of opium was by an Iranian doctor in the 800s, where he used opium as anaesthetic during surgery. Iranians' use of opium, both for medicinal and recreation purposes, was well documented in the 17th century. Over 400 years ago, Royal orders restricted its use. British colonial powers cultivated opium poppy in Iran in the 1800s and the income from opium production soon made up a huge part of then-Persia's gross national product. By 1949, there were 1.3 million regular opium users and 500 opium dens in Tehran alone. Ten years later, Iran introduced laws to prohibit the cultivation and use of opium. But by 1969, with an estimated 350,000 opium users, the law was relaxed to allow limited use and cultivation of opium for pharmaceutical purposes.

Before the Islamic Revolution in 1979, Iran cultivated up to 33,000 hectares of opium poppies, but after 1979 such cultivation was banned and completely eradicated by the end of 1980. Opium vouchers were issued to users who were given six months' grace to quit.

Iran sits on the chef opium smuggling route from Afghanistan to the West and so is swamped with drugs. Thousands of shoot-outs along this route have killed hundreds of police and many more dealers. Drug possession and trafficking laws in Iran are severe. Simple possession of 50 grams of cannabis or opium can result in a fine of USD500 and up to 50 lashes. While prison policies may be progressive, strict laws outside result in over 80,000 people being incarcerated for drug-related crimes per year. Most people with a substance use history also have a history of incarceration.

Today, Iran's rate of opium use is the highest in the world. Of 70 million Iranians, four million smoke opium, 200,000 inject it and another 100,000 inject heroin, a derivative of opium. But the sands were shifting; smoking opium was being replaced by smoking heroin, which was giving way to injecting it. A worse tide was to come: stimulants such as amphetamines had reached the shores and were about to cause more havoc than opiates.

One reason for the change in these patterns of drug use was the elaborate process required to prepare opium to be inhaled. One needed a pipe and cinders; and its use is not easily hidden. Another reason was the Taliban's crack down on poppy cultivation in Afghanistan in early 2001, making opium near impossible to find on the streets that year. That was when many users made the switch to heroin. The rising price of opium made heroin cheaper and more popular in comparison.

Heroin is still the primary choice for entrenched users in Iran. Heroin is placed on a spoon and a few drops of water and citric acid are added then the spoon is heated over a flame to dissolve the powder. Sometimes the injecting equipment would be sterilised by boiling if it's been used. If people don't clean the site on their arm where they inject, it can cause an infection.

A purer derivative of heroin is *kerack*, which was easier to prepare as it dissolves in water without having to be boiled with citric acid. However, as it was more potent, more frequent injections were required to hold off withdrawals. *Kerack* users move from inhaling to injecting faster than heroin users. In 2003, most dealers were charging USD10 for *kerack*. The use of *kerack* was extensive; it was becoming the first thing that the dealers offered new customers.

Iran's society is strictly controlled by the ruling theocratic government, especially the lives of females. The Islamic "morality police" ensure women cover their heads appropriately. If a woman failed to do so suitably, she can be arrested. Yet underneath this morally strict society, all sorts of drugs are freely available, and drug use by females is surprisingly common.

Conservatism was no protection against AIDS. For the last two decades, Iran has grappled with HIV spreading among its people. Over 18,000 registered individuals had tested positive to HIV infection, but the UN estimated the likely number was four times higher. The driving force behind Iran's HIV epidemic was multiple users on drug-filled syringes; the cause of two-thirds of the AIDS cases. In some cities, one-fifth of their drug users were infected with HIV. Among the homeless, the proportion was more; up to one-third with the dreaded infection. One of the first reports from Iran that came to my attention detailed the burden HIV infection had placed on the homeless. Bijan, the medico who presented this report at the conference, was to become an important ally.

According to most experts, opium, heroin, hashish and even alcohol were easily sourced in Tehran. Heroin was obtained from a street dealer; whereas the other ones were home-delivered. A gram of opium costs USD1, while a gram of heroin costs USD10. For comparison, 1 gram of heroin in Australia cost 30 times more than in Iran. Ecstasy use and its associated problems were taking off in Tehran along with amphetamines. Although alcohol consumption is prohibited for Muslims, others are allowed to produce their own or even bring it into the country. Armenians have their own club where they can buy and drink alcoholic beverages.

In 2004, Iran's Education Ministry disseminated AIDS awareness booklets to school kids explaining how HIV was transmitted. While they detailed the sexual activities that can spread HIV and that the use of condoms can counter the spread of HIV, it emphasized religion and family values and recommended abstaining from sex outside of marriage. It also warned against using hypodermic syringes to take illicit drugs. About one third of Iranian school students had tried alcohol and one in four university students had tried narcotics. Interestingly most students viewed users as having a mental illness and deserving of help. But while students were experimenting with drugs, the general public had poor knowledge about HIV, with negative attitudes toward HIV positive individuals prevailing among the less educated. Truck drivers and female sex workers had better knowledge about sexually transmitted infections than the youth, but their knowledge came from personal experience rather than public awareness programmes. Truck drivers had a more positive attitude to extramarital sex than youths did.

Iran's response to illegal substances has evolved over the last few decades. Detoxification was the main prong in Iran's attack in the 1970s. After the 1979 Revolution, a tough anti-drug campaign was launched. Nevertheless, heroin use shot up. Although over 100,000 users were detoxified in 1999, questions were being asked about the value of this approach as detoxification was ineffective as long-term rehabilitation. A search for a better approach, including harm reduction, began. This approach accepts the inevitability of some drug use and aims to target behaviours to reduce drug related harms to the individual and society. One of the main stays of harm reduction was the distribution of free sterile needles and syringes to people to inject illegal drugs. While Iran and other countries embraced the free needle program, the US balked at it, banning federal funds from being spent on needles. A court challenge overturned the ban briefly, but it was reinstated. The punitive and short-sighted approach by the US cost hundreds of thousands of lives and billions of dollars in health care costs.

When Iran's government reviewed its policy in 2004, it invited public health professionals and self-help groups to suggest ideas and new methods of dealing with addiction and mental health. Like many other countries, major considerations were HIV infection among people who injected and the traditional responses to drug use in general. The Ministry of Health adopted a four-pillar approach to policy, focusing on prevention, treatment, harm reduction and law enforcement. Encouragingly, the Iranian government had responded well to its AIDS crisis with very progressive and enlightened programs to the point where Iran was ahead of countries such as Australia, the UK, Canada and the USA. There was no doubt that HIV and its associated risk behaviours presented a dilemma for followers of Islam. While providing moral guidance about sexual abstinence, mutual fidelity was the cornerstone of the HIV prevention program. However, it was acknowledged that some people were unwilling or unable to follow these guidelines. Hence it was necessary to provide simple and accurate information on the importance of using condoms. Improving the negotiation and decision-making skills for their use and making them easily available were other aspects incorporated in their condom promotion program.

Iran was quick to expand their programs to stop HIV. In 2002, a widespread needle and syringe program commenced. Within a few years 50,000 people were collecting syringes from 700 locations each month, distributing a total of six million needles a year. Iran even operated a needle and syringe program in six prisons. Meanwhile methadone was being scaled up, increasing to 1,000 agencies servicing 350,000 patients per year. Ground-breaking programs saw over 10,000 people enrolled into opium maintenance programs. They considered it unfair to expect the elderly to quit opium as they developed their habit when opium use was legal. This rapid rise in coverage for HIV prevention was remarkable by world standards.

Drug use was considered a medical problem, which allowed courts to steer people to help instead of prison. Therapeutic communities operated abstinence-based groups for heroin users with 90% being referred by the courts. Critics of these communities claimed they resembled overcrowded prisons. Narcotics Anonymous and other self-help groups were popular in Iran. Even drop-in centres were established for homeless drug users. Harm reduction strategies received widespread support from senior government officials in Iran.

As early as 2005, Iran was leading the region and many western countries with its approach to HIV. Soon enough the effects of its approach were becoming obvious: Iran's rate of imprisonment dropped from being the sixth highest in the world down to the 50th highest. But in Iran's haste to promote harm reduction they had forgotten one crucial group: female drug users. And, although women could access methadone, few did. Women-only agencies were unheard of. But how many of these females there were was unknown. Women, no matter where they are, suffer more stigma for drug-taking than men do. And so they are reluctant to seek out help. Some suggested that those who engaged in sex work also injected drugs. In a small sample of female injectors, most were socially isolated and lived either alone or with another drug user. Hardly any more information was known about Iranian female users. Several attempts by researchers to recruit an adequate number of women who used drugs had failed.

Chapter 5. Establishing a Clinic for Female Drug Users

While the idea for a women's clinic was born on that day in a Tehran café in late September, 2003, it was a chance meeting with an Iranian doctor in Ljubljana, Slovenia, the previous year that had led me to Iran. Margaret and I were sitting in the middle of the audience at the 2002 International Harm Reduction Conference. The emcee, Pat O'Hare mentioned Bijan, an Iranian doctor, who had driven all night from Shiraz, in the South to Tehran in the North, a distance of more than 700 km, to obtain a visa to attend the conference. This was his first time abroad. The Iranian doctor duly stood up and took a bow. He had a rather old-fashioned camera around his neck. My first impression was that he looked like Omar Sharif, the Egyptian actor who starred in *Doctor Zhivago*, one of my mother's favourite actors.

The next day I quizzed conference attendees if they had encountered Mr Iran. Without exception they said yes, isn't he sweet, he's charming and he's pretty excited about being at this gathering. My conference presentation covered how rampant Hepatitis C was among Australian inmates, which prompted Bijan to request training for Iranian prison staff. As the conference came to a close, Bijan and I met one last time. He insisted that I ought to come to Iran. I had heard that Iran was progressive and was eager for a firsthand experience. Two outbreaks of HIV among Iranian prisoners caused a flurry of action in the 1990s. Although details of these outbreaks have escaped publication, at least a third of the inmates who were tested were infected. If true, then Iran had suffered one of the largest HIV outbreaks in prison in the world. One option mooted to deal with the outbreaks was a punitive approach where infected inmates were put to death. But a second option, the one Iran took up, was the humane approach with attempts directed at stopping HIV spreading among its prison population. This option was one to which I felt I had something to contribute.

In 1999 in Shiraz, Bijan's Persepolis Centre, a Non-Government Organisation (NGO), was one of the first to provide assistance to users in Iran. While working as a GP, he provided a room upstairs for his drug-using patients to socialise. In between patients he slipped up to the room and questioned them about what they viewed as important.

This was something unheard of then. When he moved from Shiraz to Tehran, he opened a service for users, one of the first outreach projects in Tehran with support from the United Nations. Research had pinpointed South Tehran as a hot spot with high rates of drug-related problems. His service operated two vans to provide outreach across South Tehran. Outreach is where the workers go searching for users on the street and offer needles and syringes, condoms and counselling or referral to an office-based service. Then he established a drop-in-centre to complement the mobile outreach one. One hundred clients at his drop-in centre were screened for HIV and one-third was infected, while two-thirds had Hepatitis C. They responded by scaling up advocacy activities. After nine months he and his staff were providing services to 100 clients at the drop-in centre and another 100 homeless users through outreach.

In 2002, his Persepolis NGO was a recruitment site for a methadone study to investigate if HIV related high-risk behaviour could be reduced. Clients were randomized into receiving either 40 mg versus 75 mg of methadone per day. Promising preliminary outcomes from the pilot phase prompted health authorities to implement a larger study of 785 subjects. But all the research participants were male. Then the Ministry of Health approved the first methadone program to operate at the Persepolis NGO. The program commenced with ten patients, which crept up to 50 over the next nine months and finally catered for 200 patients. All these innovative services led to Bijan being appointed as an Executive Member of the Asian Harm Reduction Network where he spoke in favour of providing treatment to women and was one of the first to do so in his Region.

In 2003, a year after his NGO opened in Tehran, the government approved the delivery of medical and social care services through community-based centres and outreach. With support from the Iran UNODC Office, the Ministry of Health and others, Persepolis developed a wide range of additional services for users and their families. Services included condom provision, voluntary HIV counselling and testing, HIV/AIDS education and social services for homeless users such as free food, tea, hairdressing, clothes and showers.

In March 2005, with the support of the Iran Medical University, Persepolis NGO opened a fourth drop-in-centre in Tehran for an additional 200 patients. With this new facility, Persepolis NGO began to deliver a wide range of services to some 800 people in Tehran, but still nearly all clients were men.

In the 2000s, drug use was on the up in the country and so were the associated harms that were a major concern. Iran had an estimated 1.7 million users in 2008; out of these, up to 300,000 may have been injecting drugs. Out of all recorded people living with HIV/AIDS in the nation, up to three quarters were using drugs; sharing used needles remained the major way to acquire HIV infection. In the first half of 2005, Persepolis NGO was a popular site for visits from the Iranian Minister of Health, high ranking law enforcement officials and delegates from the European Union as well as the United Nations. Local and international news agencies broadcasted stories of Bijan's work. More visitors came: official delegates and NGO staff from Jordan, Indonesia, Afghanistan and Sudan. Opportunities for change were being created in the Islamic Republic of Iran, both at the policy level as well as on the ground, which meant Iran could still halt its HIV epidemic. Persepolis NGO had reached a total of 3,500 users and their families in Tehran. Not only were people visiting Bijan's centre, but they were also inviting him abroad. Bijan was invited to attend the Beckley Foundation's Global Policy seminar in London in 2005.

Bijan and I met several more times; in Chiang Mia in 2003 and in Sydney in 2004. At the conference in Chiang Mai, Bijan's presentation was remarkable. He had treated over three hundred people with buprenorphine, a medicine very similar to methadone, over a three-year period. They had to procure the drug on the black market before attending his surgery for supervised dosing. Later we met in Sydney and plotted to work together. How exactly we were unsure but there was a pact between us. A conference on drug use among youth brought Bijan to Sydney and presented an opportunity to workshop three studies, two of which we managed to complete and publish. The first study was an audit of his patients. About two-thirds of his patients were using drugs and one-third were injecting. But all the users were male. He had cemented his reputation as an addiction specialist, as he had a hefty caseload of demanding patients. Opium and heroin were equally popular among his patients. About three-quarters had tried to quit drugs but most relapsed after just a few weeks. Some sought help because they were tired of using drugs, being sent to prison and running the risk of acquiring HIV infection.[5]

The second study measured Iranian doctors' knowledge of drug users and responses. All the doctors were males, in their mid-forties,

---

[5] Day et al., 2006.

who treated an average of 100 patients a week. They counselled them, provided nicotine patches and referred patients to other services, but that was it. It became obvious that this group warranted training in order to address drug addiction.[6] A third and somewhat more ambitious study, measuring not just the level of HIV infection but how fast it was spreading, was too difficult to undertake.

*

In March 2004, the year following my first visit to Iran, several Iranians colleagues including my guide and interpreter came to Australia for a drug conference that I attended. They wanted to continue our discussions about responding to prisoners, but I was still grief-stricken. I did volunteer to search for funding for the project. Over the next three years we exchanged hundreds of emails and phone calls to develop the proposal. The research program I headed up at my university aimed to encourage and support researchers and clinicians in developing countries to undertake new projects with some assistance from my team. The objective was to build their skills to carry out the work on their own. Also, when researchers and clinicians had a vested interest, they were more likely to support the project. And really who knew which particular approach was about to work in a different setting? I needed the locals to inform me what they thought might work and then rely on the research evidence to guide the proposal. My overarching research program encompassed my Iranian work.

To my surprise about this time, Iran's judiciary followed my suggestion to come to Australia and witness drug courts in action. Then Iran established drug courts as a method to divert drug users from the penal system. The Head of the Judiciary had ordered everyone working in the criminal justice system—judges, police and jailers—not to meddle with HIV programs or the people who run them. This judicial statement was the only such directive in the world. The Head of the Judiciary voiced strong support for harm reduction strategies. The executive order to all judicial authorities nationwide stipulated that HIV prevention, especially needle and syringe programs, was necessary. A statement was issued in 2005 requiring all judicial authorities in Iran to ensure that needle and syringe programs and methadone maintenance programs were not impeded through a mistaken belief that these programs were aiding criminal activities. Judges, in particular, were reminded not to

---

[6] Shakeshaft et al., 2005.

impede the programs by jailing clients. The statement was made by Seyed Mahmood Hashemi Sharoudi, Head of the Judiciary, Islamic Republic of Iran's Judicial Branch, Jan 24th 2005.

*

Initially our project was to focus on female prisoners, treat them inside and continue treatment into the community on release. Providing emergency accommodation and a crèche at the community service were also proposed. That ensured that the neediest, the terrified souls at Tehran prison, were likely to receive treatment in prison and then come to our community service when released from prison. A bus was planned to collect them at the prison gate and bring them to our centre. The plans became more and more ambitious. So what if these services were not the core component of services right on our doorstep in Sydney? Our proposed service was about to be superior to anything provided in Australia, and it was to be in Tehran, not just eight thousand miles away but in another culture with another language, a different time zone and under another religion. This elaborate proposal afforded those women a fair chance of staying out of prison. So we decided to first focus on setting up a service for females with drug problems in the community. We had to allocate funds for rent, renovations, furnishings, utilities, medical equipment, IT software, medications, diagnostics, needles and syringes, disposal of medical waste—a lesson learned earlier—and office equipment.

Each rejected proposal was refined to address additional concerns. Could we find some organisation to fund this sort of work? Was it possible to do this in Iran? Would anyone even come for treatment? Could qualified staff willing to work with sex workers even be found? What were the women's backgrounds, living situations, work and schooling like? Who introduced them to drugs? What mishaps had occurred as a result of their drug use? Had they picked up any infections? How did they fund their drug habit? Had they tried to give up drugs? Were they married? Were they forced into sex work to support their drug habits like so many others were overseas? Exactly how risky was it to sell sex in Iran? What kinds of stigma did they face? What was it like in prison in Iran, especially in terms of drugs and AIDS? What crimes had they committed? Could they have conjugal visits with their husbands like the male prisoners could with their wives? I suggested that we include transsexuals in our target group. Perhaps they could attend at night? But Bijan kept drawing me back to our original aim of helping women with drug problems.

All these questions were debated almost weekly on the phone. We had to work out what sorts of services should be provided, what kinds of staff should be employed. Would the service actually make a difference to those addicted to drugs? Those were the criteria to be judged on, not just whether they were able to quit, but whether they re-joined society, were employed or undertook study. More so, we had to be able to attribute their improvement to attending the clinic. In the world of research, you can notice a change in aspects like drug use or daily activities but to be able to attribute it to an intervention requires rigorous methodology.

It was essential that our project was sensitive to Iran's culture. The commitment to the project from both sides, Australia and Iran, had remained steadfast. I had to determine what already existed for female drug users in Iran. I rang Bijan at Moscow's airport to clarify a number of issues. He was adamant that his organisation was quite capable of managing the funds and sent some information detailing the procedure. The idea of setting up a refuge was rejected out of hand because it was thought to be insurmountable. Apparently, a local council had tried to establish a similar service but gave up after a few months.

I lamented over our failure to secure funding to Alex, my old boss. He travelled frequently for work. I asked him to try and find some funding for my Iranian clinic. He had helped start my program of international research but was lukewarm on this project. He thought we should focus on South East Asia or drug treatment in prisons. I argued I was focusing on one of our priority areas—drug treatment in prisons. He wasn't the only one hesitant about the idea of this collaboration. A senior official from the World Health Organization urged me to work with another Iranian doctor rather than Bijan. But I insisted that was the beauty of my little organisation, that I could work with whoever from the grass roots up and with people who he might not necessarily work with. He didn't seem to appreciate that I wanted to do things differently from him and his organisation. I had met the doctor he wanted me to work with, but I was happy with Bijan and we both felt a strong tie to this project

When Alex returned from overseas, he sent a simple three-line email surprising me as he had found a funder for my Iranian project.

He gave me a name and an email address. So I quickly sent this person the proposal for their consideration. This was a major breakthrough especially as Alex had tried to dissuade me from working on this project for some time. If he really had located a funder, that was a miracle. It had only been three years. Was some agency really prepared to fund a project to help this vulnerable group? I had heard that the Drosos Foundation prided itself on funding projects that were difficult to fund from traditional sources. They already had a number of projects in the Middle East, so there seemed to be a slight chance that they would fund us.

During discussions with the funder I pushed for the funding contract to be between Persepolis NGO and the funder. Then Persepolis NGO could commission my university to provide assistance with the research and development of policy and procedures manuals. The main reason for me stepping aside was that I was due to have twins in the coming months. Compounding this situation was their early arrival of ten weeks, which meant their health was very fragile and there were complications, of course. Both had jaundice and were severely underweight and one had severe respiratory distress. But I had a baby boy, Billy, and a baby girl, Georgie, at once. What a relief after trying for so many years. I sent an email to my Sydney colleagues to announce their arrival much to the amazement of some staff who had no idea that I was even pregnant. And I was not the most likely woman at work to be having a baby, let alone two! One colleague had written on my card from the office "trust you to have twins!" The babies spent one full week in intensive care. The doctor reassured me that they rarely lost a baby at this stage though there might be some problems later on from such premature births, but that they were likely to survive. My babies moved into the special care unit for nine weeks. I traipsed up there twice a day to feed and bond with them. I was producing the largest amount of milk of all the mums. The more I expressed, the more I produced. But I just had to. I had twins to feed. Although I was on six months maternity leave, I continued working on this project and a few others projects I had at that time. One project was a mission to Mongolia, which my obstetrician had banned me from joining. He reckoned the hospitals there didn't have running water. The possibility of a very early labour hadn't registered with me. I had to limit my participation to teleconferencing. During one teleconference, a person on the line questioned me about the sound of running water in the background. I had to confess that I was bathing a newborn while I was on the teleconference call.

One key stakeholder commented that this project was one of the most sensitive projects in Iran and, perhaps, in the Region. And part of it was to be based one of the most sensitive prisons in Tehran, and also in the most sensitive yard, the female yard. He also argued for their man to be the coordinator as he was likely to be more acceptable to the authorities. But I had planned to have all female staff.

Our project involved four organisations, an Iranian NGO to manage the prison component, the Persepolis NGO to host the community clinic in its building, an Iranian research centre and my research centre in Australia. The funder was well justified in asking how could I manage a project from Sydney with three organisations in Iran. I was unsure myself. The funders insisted on having an overall coordinator who was not based at the clinic but oversaw the prison program, the clinic and the research side of things. The prison doctor thought the targeted number of inmates to be recruited was too high. She was right—we had been too ambitious—we were aiming for 150 to be placed on methadone over an 18-month period. That in itself was not too much if the program was underway, but as it was the program was yet to commence and there were likely to be teething problems. So our team agreed to have a discussion with those in prison to introduce methadone and the benefits of this kind of treatment. From what we knew there would be enough need and enough interest but still we met to discuss this new treatment. While I was raising twins, the Iranians were moving the project along. After about three months, I told them about my babies and received some sweet letters and cards.

The funder was worried that international negotiations regarding Iran's nuclear plants might present a challenge to the implementation of the project. But the Iranians assured me first sanctions were likely to be imposed before a war and that those sanctions would not affect our project. But the sanctions did. They just shrugged saying that they lived in constant fear of war and so did most in the region. One person rightly noted that, if they let that stop them, they were unlikely to undertake any activity. I hadn't realised what it was like to have to carry on regardless with the threat of war in the back of your mind.

A refined proposal was submitted to the funder. Our hopes were raised a bit more. We had to satisfy the ethics committee at my university that our research was ethical. The committee were concerned that some prisoners might be coerced into treatment. They worried there might be repercussions for an interviewee if she disclosed a crime and whether we were bound to inform the authorities if someone had confessed to committing a crime. But the Iranians had carried out similar research for years without problem. According to Iranian law, researchers and medical practitioners must report criminal activity only in cases of homicide or child abuse. For other crimes, there is no obligation to inform authorities. Rather, to do so was considered a breach of professional confidentiality. Our researcher had previously collected data on criminal activity among drug using populations and had never been required to disclose any information. Our research participants needed a realistic way to lodge a complaint with our ethics committee in Sydney. So we provided international reply-paid envelopes to send complaints into the committee. My ethics committee had many concerns that we had to address to their satisfaction for the funds to be released by my university.

For our funder, this project was their first one to be based in Iran and approval from their Board was required when it next met. We were eager to hear the result and arranged for a teleconference immediately following the meeting. The Board gave the green light to fund our proposal. But first they had numerous questions and queries that had to be resolved and the finalised proposal had to be resubmitted for formal approval. This process would take another two months.

Then a contract would have to be drawn up between my university and the funder and then between my university and with each agency in Iran; the NGO to work with the Prison Department, the Persepolis Clinic, and the research centre. However, we could attend to the paperwork, while the Board's decision was pending. The funder thought the project aligned well with their priorities. But the questions they had for us were tough to answer. In fact, some answers would only be discovered during the project. They wanted to know what the social and economic profile of female drug users in Iran was like. What drugs were they taking? How would the project improve their health and family reconciliation? How would our project relate to other drug-focussed programs in Iran? And to what degree and by whom were the project activities to be coordinated with Iranian authorities? Which authorities were to be involved? Was permission needed? What was the cost of the emergency housing? By this time, we had scrapped the idea of providing emergency housing, but the other questions were fair. The funder wanted an outline of which responsibilities rested with those in

Tehran and with me in Sydney.

Although we knew little about female drug users in Iran, we knew much about females who used drugs in other countries. Women entering drug treatment were three times more likely to have major depression than untreated peers. Depression was a significant factor among those seeking treatment; it prompted them to seek treatment but also could interfere with their recovery. An essential component of our project should be a consideration of depression, with the provision of appropriate treatment.

Our funder was satisfied with our progress and pleased that we were open to discussing the ensuing problems we were facing. The funder insisted that we employ an independent accountant, and we did so immediately. They noted that Bijan was on 'extended leave.' While they were prepared to wear this situation temporarily, they were adamant that this was not in agreement with the proposal, which stated 'The Persepolis Centre Director will supervise the management of the Clinic.'

We based our clinic in the Persepolis NGO's main clinic. Bijan suggested splitting the opening times by sex. But the funder had doubts whether operating the clinic at different times was a viable solution. The funder was also demanding that we had to 'change the situation without delay. The exact requirements for such changes should be worked out in the next two months, including binding dates.' Then the funder was worried about the delay in starting the prison program. And they questioned a request for higher wages and additional equipment before the program had commenced. They thought this reflected badly on us as we had not calculated our financial planning correctly and any search for extra funding was likely to delay the project even further. However, they reassured us that they remained committed to this project and believed in the positive impact that could flow from this project for females in prisons, not only in Iran. People were hassling me about when it would start, and I could only say soon. Normally, once you received a grant, the project would be over within the year, not waiting for another year to start, and then some unknown time to actually be completed. While this project was fascinating to undertake, it was unwise career move for me.

At this point the wife of one of the key stakeholders arrived in Sydney for a conference on sexual health. She was a very warm lady and rather stylish. I vaguely remembering she struggled with our conversation in

English, but that was of no real consequence. She worked in a private clinic in Tehran that also treated transsexuals, which of course was fascinating to hear about. We dined in the gay area of Sydney and then visited Kings Cross, the red light and drug using area. She was suitably impressed with the services on offer; mobile outreach vans, syringe vending machines, a late-night harm reduction service and the supervised injecting centre, located in the middle of Kings Cross. But I was so tired I had to retire early that evening to be able to rise at 4 am to feed my twins who were now four months old. The paternal grandmother popped in most days and helped feed them and their dad helped at night.

Debate continued about whether the project coordinator should be male or female. The decision of the coordinator's gender pitted two agencies against each other. I just assumed a female was the person for this role, but the others disagreed. I had presumed she would while away the time with them in the safe room, the room where they could chat openly about their problems, including sexual ones. A male coordinator would stymie this and prevent them from removing their hejabs.

Women were mandated to wear a hejab. The Islamic revolutionary guards watch to make sure they cover their head appropriately, that they cover their hair completely. They are also obliged to wear a *Roopoosh*, a coat that hides the curves of a woman's body. The favoured dress by the government is the black *chador*, a long black cape covering from the head to the ankles. It is usually held in place by grabbing it under the chin.

The main service at our clinic was to be a methadone maintenance program. A powerful narcotic drug is dispensed to those who are physically dependent on heroin or opium. Attached to this program was to be a variety of ancillary services and, in general, more services meant better outcomes for clients. Methadone was studied thousands of times, more than any other medicine, and producing nearly always favourable outcomes. Yet methadone programs are controversial. It is a synthetic opioid that produces a slight buzz, but this means patients stay in treatment and out of trouble. Adequate doses of methadone stopped people from using heroin. Due to methadone's long half-life of about 20 hours, being the time for the effects to halve, a daily dose will suffice; whereas, heroin is typically used three times a day. The fact that methadone was legal stopped patients from committing a crime to raise the funds to pay for heroin. Also, as people drank methadone, they avoided all the injecting related problems. Methadone is a safe drug, if the guidelines are followed. The risk of overdose, both fatal and non-fatal, drops dramatically when one switches from heroin to methadone. But it had taken us so long to get moving that there were already 30 women on methadone in prison. So naturally our attention turned to the community-based clinic.

For the clinic to succeed, appropriately skilled staff members were required. Finding them was another hill to traverse. Our first priority was finding a suitable clinic director and then a coordinator. Bijan had suggested a male doctor as the clinical director. But I had envisaged an all-female team. Bijan was insistent that his nomination for the clinical director was the right one, so I acquiesced. Then some of our colleagues suggested a male coordinator was more likely to be acceptable to the Iranian authorities. There was misunderstanding and then disagreement on this point. But I was adamant that we had to have a woman in this role.

After four years of unsuccessful applications for funding, I was awarded a grant of nearly USD300,000 from a Swiss organisation in 2006. At last, we could establish a clinic for female drug users in Tehran. The workers were to include: a supervisor who was also the Persepolis Centre director, a doctor, two nurses, a social worker, a midwife, a clinical psychologist, a lawyer and an administrator. In addition, there were to be a coordinator, three researchers, an accountant and me.

This project had three components: the first was a prison-based methadone maintenance program with facilitated referral to the community-based methadone clinic, the second component. And third, there was to be a research component, a randomised controlled trial. That meant half of the sample would receive treatment immediately and half would join a waiting list for a few months and then enter treatment. The role of the coordinator was to manage all three components. She would be the lynch pin holding it all together. The person in this post would be in constant contact with all the players in Iran and with me in Sydney. Several colleagues suggested Seyah. She was a researcher but also a cardiologist and an expert on harm reduction and methadone treatment. A reasonable salary level had been allocated for all staff to ensure the best available could be recruited. It was rather surprising how low the salaries were for such highly qualified personnel. Seyah was responsible for overseeing the establishment of the clinic, and immediately set about employing the staff. We communicated through weekly teleconferences and by regular reports she emailed to me in Australia.

Seyah started in June 2007 and initially worked two days a week. It was her duty to ensure funds were disbursed to the various players and organise the itinerary for me when I came to observe and meet key people relevant to our project.

The first staff member recruited was the doctor, a lovely lady from the north of Iran. Having lived most of her life overseas, she was a little unfamiliar with Iran's drug problems. She did have a surgery and limited experience in the addiction field, but with men only. The doctor was scheduled to work six days a week supervising nursing staff, prescribing methadone, addressing other health issues and referring clients to specialists. Methadone has many advantages as an alternative to heroin and other opiates, but it must be administered under strict supervision. The doctor assessed clients, established the starting dose and the rate of increase, because too much of an increase can be fatal. A standard starting dose was 30 mg, which was increased by 5 mg, twice a week, until the client was stabilised. The client had to be closely supervised for three months and the dose adjusted accordingly. Consuming depressant type drugs, like alcohol or benzodiazepines on top of methadone could be life-threatening. As so few female heroin users had any experience of receiving drug treatment, they were clueless as what to expect and what was expected from them.

A strong team of researchers on the ground was essential. The team comprised three Iranian researchers; one senior and two research assistants. The senior researcher identified two research assistants and ran a workshop to train them up on the techniques to be used. Their tasks included interviewing each woman after a few weeks of attendance and then again after six months to determine any changes. They also carried out individual in-depth interviews and focus groups on a variety of topics. The research assistants were young, naïve girls who were shocked to learn about the topics they were to study. Other research duties were entering data on the computer and checking for any inconsistencies.

Our primary aim was to attract women and keep them in our care. One key outcome was their use of heroin or opiates. If treatment worked, then heroin use should decrease within a few months. We had edited the questionnaire between us; it was translated into Farsi for training the research assistants and for their use of it and should have been translated back to English to examine how it compared to the original version. Somehow this didn't happen. Also, several questions I wanted to include were too sensitive, while others specific to Iran's drug culture warranted inclusion.

The World Health Organization has classified a whole range of diseases. We used the ICD10—the international classification of diseases used for general epidemiological and many health management purposes. Our first line of inquiry was whether these people were dependent on drugs. For these criteria to be met, three or more manifestations had to occur together for at least one month; otherwise, they had to have occurred together repeatedly within a twelve-month period.

*

Marriage is held in high regard in Iran. Iranians can enter into a temporary marriage. Men view some photos of potential brides and choose one to marry. The marriage can last from one hour to ninety-nine years. In the temporary marriage, it is necessary to determine the appropriate duration and gift, *mehrieh*, or the marriage would be annulled. Surprisingly, a temporary marriage was not just about sex; it was also for *mahram,* where the woman could reveal her body and hair in front of her husband or his relatives. The husband should not be away from his wife for more than four months at a time. The wife can state in the contract that she doesn't want to have intercourse, just the other benefits. Young girls can enter a temporary marriage, but the duration of marriage should be extended until the girl was old enough to enjoy sex. If a man and woman were temporarily married, they could not inherit from each other, but any offspring could inherit from their parents. The man was not obliged to support the woman financially, even if she became pregnant. They could be married on a permanent basis, but first they should terminate the temporary marriage. A woman cannot have sex with another male while in a temporary marriage, but a man can have sex with his other wives. Men can have four permanent wives and any number of temporary wives, simultaneously. When a woman ends a marriage, whether it was a temporary or permanent one, she must not marry again for four months and ten days, a period known as *eddeh*. These marriages occur in the Shiite branch of Islam, not the Sunni branch.

Chapter 6. The Opening of the Women's Clinic

July 30th 2007 was a momentous day—the opening of our clinic for women seeking drug treatment in Iran. From my office in Sydney, I eagerly inquired how the first day unfolded. Would anyone come along? What kind of person would come? And if they came, would they stay? Iran was six and a half hours behind Sydney, so we had to wait until mid-afternoon the next day to hear how the first day went. I needn't have worried—it did not take long for them to meander into our clinic.

Our host centre, the Persepolis NGO, was located near the Azim-Abad Castle, a 3,500-year-old ruin in Shoosh Square. During the past decade, Afghan refugees had settled in the area and unemployment was high among the youth. Street peddlers sold flowers, watches, newspapers, chewing gum, tea, chocolates, clothes and toys. Our building was a blue cement two storey one. The outside of the building was ordinary looking, perfect for a controversial service. The doorway fronted onto a very busy road with a bus stop almost at the door and a taxi rank just a few metres along. Nearby the underground metro ran. The heavy pedestrian traffic outside was another important aspect that would allow our clients to blend into the hustle and bustle on the busy street. Shoosh Square was also home to a large street drug scene.

It was an exciting time when the first few in-depth interviews had occurred. The senior researcher rang me, declaring that the research had begun and she read out some interviews over the phone. The assistants enjoyed their jobs as the clients appreciated being heard, being studied and being cared about. A pleasant interview process would aid in relocating interviewees down the track, though a few thought the interview was long and boring. The senior researcher and I would analyse the results together. Our study examined benchmarks of one's drug use, such as their age of drug initiation and of commencement of daily drug use. These benchmarks indicated certain aspects about a user's life. On average, members of our group were 22 years old when they first used an illegal drug. But this concealed the fact that some first used when they were just 10 years old, while others did not begin until they were 52 years old. Half of our group were married, mostly for the first time, but some were on their second marriage. Although divorce had quite a stigma attached to it, many were divorced or separated.

Alongside the interviews, blood and urine samples were collected and tested for HIV and Hepatitis C, and for traces of heroin, respectively. With all the delays we experienced, the HIV test kits were about to expire, and we had too many to use before they would expire. I urged the researcher to give the kits to another service rather than waste them. We tried to ring each other to discuss this and other matters but kept missing each other. After two weeks the interviewers had surveyed 18 women. It was surprising that the research was rolling on smoothly. Then when our senior researcher announced she was leaving Iran to study abroad, I was disheartened. Although she believed she could continue her job from abroad. I was reluctant to add another country into the mix, as there would surely be some repercussions for the research. And then the doctor had left too, but a replacement was soon located for her.

A few clients complained about the interview being too long, with some refusing to do it. It was time for a sweetener. The supervisor proposed handing out coupons that could be exchanged for food or toys. While giving coupons was a swell idea, it required persuading a shopkeeper to cooperate with the scheme, and a shop where they wanted to use their coupons.

*

It would be six years before I had the chance to make my second visit to Iran, and two years after the clinic opened. Stepping inside the door of the clinic was a strange experience. I had seen photos and heard reports, but still I was unprepared for the poor presentation of the clinic. My high hopes gave way to much disappointment. Inside the front door was a staircase, which was pretty grotty, dim and steep. The middle of each step was worn away from previous visitors over the years. Halfway up the staircase on the landing was a bathroom with a squat toilet and everything in it was filthy. The floor was disgusting, and the tiny room stank. A dirty rag hanged down in front of a mirror on the wall, which hid a two-way mirror that allowed staff to observe a urine sample being given. This was to ensure the sample was fresh as opposed to being a stored one from another person that would test negative to drugs.

Up the second flight of stairs there were doorways on both sides of the staircase. On the right side was the administration room, an accountant in his room and a meeting room. Behind the administration room was a small kitchen that staff used to make tea and food for themselves and the clients. Across the stairwell was the methadone room with a metal hatch in the wall that folded down allowing methadone to be passed to the patient to consume it under supervision. Off this room was a section where a nurse would hand out "harm reduction packages" containing needles, syringes and condoms, all wrapped in newspaper. These packages looked like a serve of fish and chips you might buy in an English coastal town.

I came upon the safe room, along the dingy corridor, a women's only space where they could sit and talk and take off their hejabs. I was overwhelmed by the smell of fresh paint. They had just painted this room for my visit. It seemed longer than the other rooms but actually it was just because it had a table in the middle of it and a telly at the other end. All the walls were bare. Over the next few days as the paint dried, the posters and decorations went back up and softened the stark walls somewhat. There were a few kids' chairs in the corner and some books, but apart from that, that was it. I asked about making the place more welcoming. What had happened to the funds to decorate the place? I had specifically set funds aside for decorating the rooms, so they would be very welcoming. I had imagined a harem style décor, with long flowing hangings and soft cushions on the floor. Instead, straight-backed wooden chairs fringed a huge table turning the room into a cold boardroom. I had offered to buy a coffee machine, but the Iranians preferred to drink tea.

I wanted to have a proper poke around the clinic having seen just a few rooms and there were more to inspect. I tried to make small talk with the staff, but they seemed busy with their own conversations. Just then Bijan's father-in-law came in. At first, I didn't recognise him as it had been six years since I last saw him and then just for one evening. He recognised me though and joked about our last meeting when he argued with his wife.

Most rooms opened onto a long corridor that ran along the outside of the building. The corridor was exposed to the elements, which made traversing from room to room unpleasant in winter. The first room had the doctor sitting just inside the door looking very officious and next to her was the nurses' station where they were dispensing methadone through the hatch to the other side. There was a safe here as the methadone had to be kept under lock and key as it was such a valuable commodity on the black market. Next door was the manager's room. She had several roles; supervising staff, recording stats and overseeing the receipt of the methadone and return of the empty bottles. Next along the corridor were the rooms for the midwife, the psychologist and the safe room where clients would watch TV, DVD movies and educational films about harm reduction.

Apparently, the recruitment of nurses was difficult at this time in Iran. They were hopeful that two suitable candidates would be found soon. During the orientation phase, women who were already clients of the Persepolis Clinic joined the women's clinic. This allowed for continuity of care for those enrolled at the main clinic and also gave staff an opportunity to orientate themselves to this new work with a light patient load. I predicted that finding the right staff would be a challenge, so extra funds had been allocated for advertising the various positions. It was the coordinator's job along with the director to recruit staff. With so few workers having had any experience of working with females with drug problems in Iran, it took a considerable time to reach full staffing levels.

Each new client underwent an extensive assessment. After we became more acquainted with each client, the staff inquired more about their lives, their use of drugs, their family and what support they had—and perhaps most importantly what they perceived as their main problem, which surprisingly was not their drug use.

Negotiations were still progressing with prison officials about the project. Our proposal specified a randomised trial design. While this approach was scientifically very rigorous, it was unpopular with staff and clients equally. They disliked having some arbitrary mechanism decide which patients received treatment or not. A move away from this design would have serious consequences for the research. If a study used a randomly selected sample, then any effect could be attributed to the treatment or intervention, but if the sample was selected according to the doctor's opinion, then the reason for any effect could not be attributed to the treatment. Maybe new users were not yet so entrenched in the heroin lifestyle and would improve anyway. Or maybe old users were unlikely to improve any time soon. Serious researchers push for randomised trials whenever possible, especially if a new drug was being trialled or a proven drug was introduced into a new setting or with a new client group, like ours. Another concern was about the clients who might be released early from prison. The prison staff wanted to wait to find out a woman's release date before enrolling her in the research. I was unaware of all the available options to solve the problem. Eventually, it was agreed that the doctor would decide which clients would go on methadone. And with that decision our chance to do a randomised trial disappeared.

Unfortunately, there were still no nurses employed at the clinic. Some staff thought the reason may be related to the location, but the coordinator thought differently, as there were some good workers on board who could cope with travelling to the clinic. Although the manager had no idea why it was difficult to recruit nurses, she was confident she could employ some soon. The positions were advertised in the newspapers many times. At last, a nurse who graduated about three years ago joined us. She had some experience with substance users and with psychiatric patients and was enthusiastic about her new position at the clinic. She harboured some reservations as the building appeared run down and dirty and wondered if some prospective clients were likely to be put off.

One of the first clients to hesitantly step through our front door was young, using drugs and pregnant. Zahra appeared so youthful, 18 years old at the most and was very pregnant. Zahra was a bright and bubbly girl, but just a girl. Her white dress made her look angelic. When she removed her hejab, her long shiny black hair tumbled down around her softly made up face. Her voice revealed excellent schooling. Zahra was an unusual first client, with most others being twice her age. This suggested she might have had an unusual route into using drugs, so I was intrigued to hear how she found her way to us. Most waited until a tragedy occurred before seeking help. Zahra's life away from us, was unimaginable for me. Was she pacing the street scoring drugs in her condition? How was she financing her drug habit? Who was supporting her? Her *Roopoosh* was daringly short, revealing tanned legs. She almost seemed unharmed by her drug use, not at all sleep deprived.

After a few weeks of attendance, she accepted an invitation to be part of a focus group. Zahra removed her hejab to fiddle with her black hair and then recovered her hair in a slightly different style. Her teeth looked strong and healthy. And surprisingly it was her teeth that led her to become tangled up in drugs. At 16 she had an excruciating toothache, so her uncle gave her some opium. He placed a small piece of opium in a glass of hot black tea and stirred it until it dissolved. She sipped the tea. Of course, it numbed her discomfort but it was so euphoric she continued using it. Others in her family were also opium users. She came from Shiraz, home of the poet Hafez. The girl's story toppled out of her. She twisted her hair around her fingers and played with her hejab. As her story was being interpreted, I trailed a few sentences behind the others. A serious complication with her pregnancy was diagnosed by a doctor at five months. The baby had a hole in the heart and was unlikely to survive. The doctor recommended she have a termination, a decision not taken lightly in Iran. She disagreed with the diagnosis and continued with the pregnancy. How could she disagree? He didn't say there was a high chance of having this condition; he said the baby's heart had a hole. Today she was at the seventh month mark, the beginning of her third trimester. I had an inkling how she felt. Two years previously my twins had been born with complications at seven months. They were in hospital for ten weeks with one week in the intensive care unit.

Her prescribed amount of methadone was unlikely to be adequate for her to stay away from heroin or opium. Not only was it too low, but she was deliberately reducing her dose to come off completely. A ripple of shock waves flowed around the group as this admission potentially placed her and the baby in danger. Conversations ricocheted around the circle of concerned listeners. Staff urged her to consider her baby. The interpreter was chastising her for this rash decision. Another suggested we ask why she was doing this. 'I won't be able to manage the bus ride here with my baby; it takes me an hour,' she complained. She was adamant she would taper her dose and cease therapy all together. One after the next we argued with her that this was a foolish move, not the best course of action. Solutions were put to her; couldn't a relative mind the baby while she made the trip here? What about the father, what was he doing? Or her mother, was she nearby and able to help?

It is imperative that pregnant heroin users are placed on methadone throughout their pregnancy. Indeed, in some places pregnant heroin users are often the exceptions who can receive methadone, when no one else can. Zahra lived with her husband's family and thought her mother-in-law would come to realise her problem with drugs, if she stayed on methadone. The interpreter, a staff member and I broke away from the circle to have an urgent discussion among ourselves. I wondered whether the midwife could visit her and deliver her methadone, perhaps a week's supply at once. But home delivery of methadone was against policy. I then pursued a different angle.

Could the young girl be allowed to collect several days' doses at a time? I knew clients at private clinics in Iran were permitted to take home several doses but only after months of adherence to the rules. But, no, that was not an option either. I was very concerned about the girl. If she ceased methadone treatment, she would without doubt resume heroin use. Using heroin when you're pregnant can seriously affect the baby; there was an increased risk of miscarriage and a baby will go through withdrawals if it becomes dependent on heroin from the mother's blood supply. Also, it was unknown how serious the hole in the baby's heart was and how she would react. We all hoped we could convince her to remain in treatment.

If her husband used drugs but was not in treatment, then how was she expected to abstain? His use of drugs might even depend on her continuing drug use. I tried to ask about the girl's husband, but the discussion was racing ahead and onto another issue. Patiently I waited until there was a space for my question.

The interpreter turned and said 'Yes, he was a user, but he was in treatment elsewhere and a bit closer to home.'

I had to know why she wasn't attending there. The girl's speech was like a machine gun leaving the interpreter struggling to keep pace. While we were huddled around this poor girl listening to her predicament, someone jumped up and offered tea to everyone. It was one of the client's jobs to serve tea. This was a welcomed break for the circle of listeners who had formed around her. One woman lit a cigarette while another went to the toilet. Someone else disappeared and then reappeared with some biscuits and fruit. I joked that it was no wonder all the women came here if they were given such treats. But they hinted it was because I was there, normally there were no biscuits and no fruit. So we sat and drank our tea and looked at the poor girl, all wondering what her fate would be.

Zahra's immediate issue was her pregnancy. The Iranians were adamant that they should employ a midwife on the staff. I was unsure because the role of a midwife differed in Iran. Her job was more about sexual health rather than delivering babies. The midwife had many questions about her role when we employed her. Having worked in the field for two years, she was well acquainted with female sexual health issues, for example, family planning, sexually acquired infections and HIV education. But the midwife had little experience with females who used drugs and was apprehensive about the cases she would be assigned. Also, her husband had expressed his disapproval about the job as it might reflect badly on her to be mixing with our clientele. Demand for the midwife's services was high from day one. The midwife was an elderly lady, with much life experience, before and after the Revolution. She was also very religious and made sure her work followed the Koran as close as possible. The midwife had been called on to care for this girl. The midwife had seen the teenager in her room, which was simple yet comfortable, and had put the girl at ease. If necessary, she would refer this girl to a specialist. She counselled her about safe sex, vaginal hygiene and common infections.

I was drawn to the midwife when we first met. The back wall of her examination room was blue, and the side walls were white. As we entered, she rose from her desk, which was situated in one corner. An examination couch was against the wall on the far side of the room above which was a medicine cupboard with all sorts of ointments and medications that Iranian midwives can prescribe. Basically, she investigated female sexual health. I never quite understood how this didn't overlap with the doctor's work, but it didn't even though she was able to prescribe medication.

The interpreter motioned for us to resume our positions to hear the remainder of Zahra's story. She had fallen for a magic bullet cure for her addiction and underwent a radical form of drug treatment. The "doctors" claimed that they would put her to sleep and when she woke she would be cured. Who wouldn't want to be rid of a drug habit magically and immediately? The procedure was ultra-rapid opiate detoxification. The girl was given a general anaesthetic and then pumped full of naltrexone, an anti-heroin drug that displaces heroin from the body to bring on withdrawals. She did not feel any pain as she was anaesthetised and unconscious for 24 hours. On awakening she received intramuscular injections, of what she was unsure. So she had supposedly become free of opiates. If she took a narcotic such as heroin or opium, she would respond like she had never taken it before and most likely overdose. This treatment was similar to what ambulance workers administer to a person who has overdosed on heroin. I couldn't believe this form of shoddy treatment had surfaced in Iran. Australia had its own experience of it back in the 1990s when this form of "treatment" graced the cover of a magazine. The headline was I WENT TO SLEEP A JUNKIE AND WOKE UP CURED. But, by the very fact Zahra was sitting here looking for treatment, it meant the magic bullet had missed its mark.

Then she spoke of another attempt to become drug-free, how she had dirty blood taken from her back. I had to stop the interpreter to clarify this point. This time she was referring to cupping, an old Greek remedy, and I guessed an Iranian one, too, where a heated cup was pushed onto one's back and held there while the flesh and toxins were drawn up. I couldn't fathom how this procedure would cure an addiction to heroin. Zahra underwent this procedure not once but multiple times. After three days, she was back using drugs. The treatment cost USD250, the equivalent of the average monthly salary for a professional in Iran. Zahra was desperate to beat her heroin addiction, but was poorly informed of the various modalities available.

Again, our circle around her broke away for another discussion among ourselves. The dilemma that faced me was how much input should I have in this girl's treatment? Should I allow the staff to deal with this problem in their own way? Or should I interfere and assert some special position as a supervisor, chief investigator or because I was more experienced? I was being tested as to whether I trusted the staff and it was a very uncomfortable decision to make.

This time I asked the coordinator to come with me for a private discussion. I required reassurance that she knew what to do, again assuming the girl would follow our recommendation. Immediately she convinced me of her competence and that Zahra was to be urged to remain in methadone treatment. Now, if only we could convince Zahra to listen. As I left the room, the coordinator approached Zahra to explain the benefits of this form of substitution treatment, without having to translate it for me. An appointment for organised for Zahra to consult the doctor and discuss her treatment.

The social worker completed a registration form for the newcomers. No one seemed to object. In other countries, clients refuse to provide personal details and complex ID codes have to be concocted to hide the identity of the person. But here in grotty South Tehran they felt comfortable enough to furnish very personal details. This simple fact made us realise that we were able to build a rapport with them soon after they had arrived.

Clients were asked many questions when they registered. Like most Iranians, they were predominantly Persian. A few were Azeri, coming from Azerbaijan and spoke Turkish while others were Balouch, descendants of Turkmen weavers who were among the poorest in the country. About half had been married and about a quarter was on their second marriage. Some had been divorced or separated from their husbands. Most were in their thirties, though the youngest was 18 and the oldest was close to 60. Two in three had attended high school and about one in four had attended college to do a diploma or degree. But one in four women had skipped school altogether. One regretted having no schooling and even now longed to attend school. I made mention of her desire to Bijan to explore this opportunity for her.

A few women were attending the Persepolis NGO before we opened the clinic. But they were attending what was essentially a men's clinic with over 200 men and just a smattering of females. So it was impossible to provide any special care for women when they were so outnumbered by men. But word had got out that they were welcome and there were female staff to serve them. A few heard about us while they were in prison or in police custody, which encouraged us as it indicated support in the broader community.

Most people with a serious drug problem find it impossible to hold on to a job and our clients were the same. The vast majority was jobless and half had no skills that would enable them to secure a job. This skills shortage was an area that the workers could address. Clients came from all different walks of life; they were hairdressers, weavers and some did crocheting. And predictably most had children, though not always in their care. Indeed, custody of children was one issue our lawyer could assist with. The vast majority lived in their own flat, but some were living with relatives or were homeless.

Recovery from addiction was our core business. These women were vulnerable to assault. One in four had been attacked in the last year and mainly at the hands of their partner or a family member. This group had experienced some horrific events such as having direct combat experience in a war, being involved in a life-threatening accident, witnessing someone die or be badly injured. Very few reported being raped before the age of 16, while a few more reported this had occurred thereafter. We explored whether anyone had suffered Post Traumatic Stress Disorder, a severe anxiety response to a very disturbing event. And to be expected they had felt terrified or helpless by these adverse events, which resulted in intrusive thoughts in their daily lives.

*

In the clinic's large meeting room, I finally met the supervisor, who had come in especially today. I had heard much about him, good mostly from Bijan. He was busy, working two jobs. He had a bushy beard, was a little dishevelled and looked tired. I had heard conflicting reports about whether he spoke English. A colleague who I met in Poland two months earlier told me she spoke to him in English. Yet when we met, we needed an interpreter. He worked at the men's clinic before our clinic opened, but this was his first experience of working with females.

On the occasions he ventured into the safe room to converse with those there, he left thinking they preferred to talk to the female staff. There were some complaints about bad tempered staff, but he told me it was important to keep control. Clients misinterpreted strictness for bad temper. I guessed this was an area where staff can be trained how to deal with difficult clients without losing it. He attempted to encourage the male relatives of female clients to also attend so the women would continue attending.

Meeting and chatting with the clients provided an incredible insight into their lives and their families. Today's discussion topic was drugs, and Mona was invited to join us and she acquiesced. Oddly, her face appeared much younger than her 40 years. Her large lips were enlarged with deep purple lipstick. Her foundation, which was caked on, appeared to be just touched up rather than applied fresh daily. Mona's plump body was cloaked in dark clothes, as nearly all the clients wore. Large sunglasses hid her eyes. There was a faint acidic smell around her. She brought her photo album to show me, which pleased me as she had seemed quite aloof usually. Later, I realised I had misinterpreted her depression as aloofness. On many occasions, she plonked herself next to me. I didn't mind as I thought under different circumstances we might have been friends.

We all filed into the safe room while those who were not part of the session left. The interpreter asked Mona to describe her introduction to drugs. She nodded and seemed pleased to have an audience. She was Persian and a proud one. Persians are the dominant group in Iran, making up over half of the population. Her upbringing was ordinary by her account. Mona breezed through school and expected to study at university. As she spoke, I could see she was educated as the interpreter kept raising her eyebrows when relaying her eloquent story. Later she confirmed that she was impressed with Mona's command of the language. At the age of 24 Mona was studying for a science degree, which was also when she consumed her first alcoholic drink. After graduating, she secured a position in her field and seemed content. Her job paid her handsomely. Her colleagues were often playful, mucking around at work and seemed secretive about something or other. So she confronted them as to why they acted so silly. One admitted they were using opium and a colleague shared some with her showing her how to smoke it. And that was her introduction to drugs, at the age of 28. For five years she puffed away at opium and without too many hassles, but then her use nosedived out of control, like a kite that had lost its wind.

At the end of a very busy week, the boss told Mona to find some other place to get stoned. Initially her savings kept her cocooned in a narcotic haze, but when she had churned through them, she leant on her husband. Without any income, she stole from shops, handbags on the bus; just petty crime to feed her habit. From opium she moved on to sniffing heroin. But she was adamant: she never shot up drugs. Heroin was dirt cheap in Tehran, about USD6 a gram, which could last a user from a day up to a week. At the peak of her habit she stayed up all night taking drugs and slept all day. Along with the heroin, she drank; a lethal combination as both drugs can suppress one's breathing causing one to overdose and die.

As with any drug scene there were rituals peculiar to Iran. It was customary for a dealer to provide the first shot of heroin for free, according to Mona. Experienced drug users or *malaghehdar* were paid in either money or drugs if they helped or actually injected someone. The *malaghehdar* prepared the drugs in a spoon from which several people drew up their share of the drugs. The dealer had spare injecting equipment, most likely used and possibly infected, for anyone and everyone to use. Some people used a *malaghehdar* because they were afraid to carry syringes on their person or they needed assistance to find a vein or to even inject. 'When a user was in withdrawal, they wanted their hit of heroin immediately,' said Mona. Guys tended to shoot up in public places like parks, under bridges and in alleyways, but women preferred to inject at home or in another user's house.

Mona was married and this dictated her position when a mixed group of people shot up drugs together. When a woman injected with men, she injected first if she was the sister of one of the guys. But she was relegated to last position if she was the wife of a guy in the group or if she was a sex worker.

I found this discriminating nature of the scene intriguing. The coordinator acknowledged that in this scenario, wives and sex workers most likely received a smaller amount of drugs which actually protected them from overdosing. However, by injecting last on the Conga line of syringe-sharing, their risk of catching HIV or hepatitis increased. The coordinator sat back to consider which position was preferable. Was it better to overdose or to pick up an infection? Others debated which infection, as some thought it didn't matter if you got Hepatitis C but as for HIV you wouldn't want that. But if you went first and overdosed then surely someone would tend to you as you were the first to drop? Our discussion on the relative merits of being first versus being last in the injecting line was interrupted by a knock at the door. The waitress came in and we broke off our discussion for refreshments.

After tea Mona provided more details of the woman's role in the drug scene. She explained that females who injected were more likely to share syringes than males because they required assistance to procure and prepare the drugs males injection. And they also often relied on others for a covert place to inject. Mona indicated that, although syringes can be bought at pharmacists for a small price, users shared syringes because a shared injection implied belonging to a group. And in the case of sharing someone else's syringe in a mixed group, this pleasure can even be sexual in nature.

When Mona came to us, she had never confided in anyone about the extent of her drug habit even though her life was crippled from it. She lost any control she had over her drug use; she oscillated from being stoned and overdosing to experiencing menacing drug withdrawals. To relieve her symptoms, she used again. By the time she fronted up, she was locked in this pattern of intoxication and withdrawal for 14 years. At this point she started sobbing uncontrollably. The circle broke up and moved away to give her some space. A cigarette was offered to her then a lighter was flicked on. The group was silenced by her admission. To have used drugs for 14 years would undoubted meant she engaged in numerous activities, probably put herself in danger, and had many traumatic events that would have changed her forever. In fact, she was later diagnosed as having Post Traumatic Stress Disorder. The interpreter's eye caught mine; and with her one raised eyebrow questioned whether we should continue this line of inquiry. I shrugged and left it up to her to decide while I went to the kitchen to get some water.

At the peak of her habit she overdosed nearly every other day, which was somewhat unusual for someone who mainly sniffed heroin. I had to ask if this was when she was injecting—even though she denied injecting—the interpreter confirmed it was indeed the case.

'I realised I might not live very long if I kept overdosing,' Mona said. 'One of my friends died right in my lounge room, while I was in the bathroom. I didn't want to live but I didn't want to die, well not from drugs. I had two friends, but they were a waste of time. And I hate my husband. I'm so desperately unhappy in my marriage. I want out. I wish he would die.' This provoked a resounding yes from the group. Many clients had fractured relationships with family members.

For an assessment of Mona's mental state, our psychologist administered the Beck Depression Inventory; a collection of 21 questions that measured the intensity, severity and depth of depression in patients. The worst possible score was 63, and a score between 30 and 63 meant a diagnosis of being severely depressed. Mona scored 51, well into the severely depressed zone. Mona complained that she was so miserable that it was unbearable. She expected to stuff up everything, felt a total failure as a person and felt guilty constantly. She lost confidence in herself and criticized herself for all her faults. She wanted to kill herself and felt like crying but could do neither. All these attributes were defining characteristics of severe depression. Over the last year Mona was physically assaulted by an acquaintance. She was bashed, slapped or kicked on 20 separate occasions last year. Mona was left scared, upset and, whenever she remembered it, her body reacted. Mona was caught up in a war, probably the Iran-Iraq war and thought she might be suffering Post Traumatic Stress Disorder.

*

The next time she sauntered in when I was there, she chain-smoked cigarettes all day long. She had to consult several staff immediately; the psychologist, the doctor and the lawyer. She was high on the list of priorities for the lawyer who worked just one day a week. The lawyer came highly recommended, as she had topped her class at law school. In her role, she provided legal advice to the clients. Mona's pleaded for assistance to apply for a divorce. Many clients were in relationships that hindered their recovery. If their partner was an addict, there was nil chance of remaining abstinent from drugs. Mona, like many, was unaware of her legal rights. Some were illiterate and most were ignorant of the law—so much so the lawyer ran a training session and explained their rights on issues concerned with their family and children. I asked Mona if the lawyer had helped her yet, but she shook her head. This made no sense so I pursued it further before she claimed that it was unclear whether the lawyer would help her. Then I met the lawyer to discuss Mona's case to clarify the situation. The lawyer wanted our social worker to escort Mona to court. I objected. I expected this to be one of our lawyer's duties.

I even went over the job description with the lawyer: "The clinic will employ a lawyer to attend one day each week to provide advice to clients on legal issues and offer legal representation when appropriate."

I blamed the lawyer and the lawyer blamed Mona. We disagreed on what was "appropriate." I couldn't seem to resolve this to my satisfaction. The court would appoint a lawyer, she insisted, if Mona can't afford one. But I anticipated our lawyer would accompany Mona to court and apply for a divorce for her. I made a mental note to bring this up with management later.

When the lawyer refused to help Mona's case, I felt we had let her down. I toyed with the idea of asking her to come for cup of tea outside, but the interpreter would be required and she was unlikely to agree. I suspected that I probably shouldn't be socialising with our clients in the back streets of South Tehran. I couldn't have visited her home as she lived with a violent husband; plus, I had urged the staff not to do this. So I had to be satisfied with chatting with her in the safe room.

As the group broke up, and I slipped out to go to toilet, Mona followed me and tried to explain something to me through the door, but of course I couldn't understand her. She stood outside the toilet repeating the same foreign words that seemed rather important. I called out the interpreter's name as a solution to this pickle, an indication that a go between was essential, but when I came out, she had left for the day. And I was left wondering what was so important to her.

When the lawyer was going on maternity leave in 2009, the director planned to leave the post vacant. He felt that role of a lawyer was limited and not the most ideal way to spend that amount of money. His preference was to hire more nurses or even employ a psychiatrist. He felt strongly that they were suffering in this area and deserved expert help. The call for a psychiatrist became more apparent every day. Some clients were so severely depressed that their ability to recover was compromised.

The administrator came in and announced it was lunchtime. She went on to say that the pizza maker had been instructed to use high quality ingredients as there was a guest from overseas. She was expecting a baby in three months. I took a guess and brought a pink jumpsuit for her baby; luckily, she was expecting a girl. I was starving and honoured in equal measures to be dining with the staff. It seemed strange to be eating such an American signature dish, pizza and coke, in Iran of all places. A few others joined us as we sat around a large table; the accountant, the two nurses and two secretaries. I sat next to the interpreter so we could check what remained to do that afternoon. Soon the space would be overrun by male clients, so, if we had any desire to do more interviews, we had to hurry. Also, the staff we employed would leave soon, so today we had to decide if there was anyone who we had to speak with.

In any country, including Iran, drug-addicted women have special needs. As most were mothers, they required some childcare assistance to attend treatment. This presented a dilemma for us: should we allow clients to bring their children here? While it was not an ideal setting for children to frequent, we knew if the mother couldn't leave the child with someone then she would be unable to come along if children were barred. Further, many women were fearful, and rightly so, that their children might be removed from them if they were perceived to be unable to care for them. In all probability, the husband used drugs as well, and perhaps her sons, too. It could be in his interest for his wife to use drugs so she doesn't nag him to stop him using, and she can even aid his drug use by engaging in petty crime or sex work. While money and drugs were usually split between a husband and a wife, when they both had drug habits to feed, it was not always an equal split.

Research suggested females tended to have more serious drug problems than men. They were more likely experience unemployment, depression, anxiety and medical problems and to suffer a drug-related death. Iranian females also experienced greater stigmatisation than males did and were reluctant to seek treatment, which was why very little was known about them. One study in Iran had set out to recruit female drug users but managed to enrol only four out of the 100 they sought. Their plans to hold focus groups were shelved when their target group was too nervous to partake. A women-only service could enable a better rapport to be developed which, in turn, could foster research.

So how does one get caught up in drugs? A common myth about becoming involved in drugs is that some stranger pushes drugs onto an unsuspecting victim. If only drug use could be attributed to something beyond an individual's control. But, in reality, drug initiation results from one's desire to experiment, to escape their lives, as a way to cope or just to have fun. While the reasons for initiation into drugs may vary from person to person, most people have basically chosen to take drugs. The other aspect that many don't realise or perhaps want to acknowledge is that taking drugs can be pleasurable. Humans have sought psychotropic or mood-altering states for centuries. The difference between having a glass of wine with dinner and having a joint or even a shot of heroin rests in the legality of the drug and not in the effects, as they are all mood altering.

Reasons our clients gave for beginning their drug use careers were: my partner, my sibling or even my parent took drugs; or it was about 'enjoying drugs.' Other reasons cited were to 'relieve physical pain' and 'forget family problems.' One woman said 'I married a man against my father's wishes, and we had two kids. When we divorced, my parents rejected me and my kids and so to forget my problems, I turned to drugs.'

Of the first 30 users who climbed our stairs seeking assistance, just a few had come from prison. One client lived a long way away and once she realised that the daily commute would be problematic, she left. Some clients were very young with severe problems from injecting drugs and had resorted to petty crime. The workers were quite shocked to meet so many women with such severe drug problems. While they should have been familiar from their work with men, they still found themselves in uncharted territory. Almost half of those who came along reckoned that they were introduced to drugs by their partner, while a third attributed their introduction to a friend. In fact, only one in 20 blamed a stranger for their initiation to drugs. Another piece of evidence that debunked the strangers' role in drug initiation was that most clients had their first hit at home or at a friend's place.

Another common idea about drugs is the gateway theory. According to this belief if someone begins with cannabis then they will move onto heroin and become dependent. But these women hadn't followed that path, with two out of every three having started out using opium, and then moved onto heroin. And they were rather late in their drug initiation, with most commencing in their early twenties. It would be another six years, on average, for them to inject drugs, if they did at all.

As one would expect most users had first consumed drugs by smoking, given that they were using opium. Very few people begin by injecting drugs. Although some had injected, most were not doing so when they sought help. Like most drug users, they were using an assortment of drugs.

To target drug treatment appropriately, it was imperative to determine the primary drug. A resounding majority reported it to be heroin, opium or morphine. This was not only their drug of choice, but it was the drug causing the most problems. This confirmed our strategy of offering methadone, the heroin substitute. However, a few others used amphetamines and help for them was also essential. Amphetamines treatment is less well developed, in comparison to those for heroin users.

*

The next client we spoke to in-depth was Maryam. Her black crocheted shawl caught my eye immediately. Clutching her large tan vinyl handbag, she reminded me of my grandmother; she probably was somebody's grandmother. The first thing she did was pinch my cheek and hard, just like my granny did. As she was much more senior than the others, she stood out. And like many, she was quite plump. I guessed she was in her mid- or even late 50s, but it seemed impolite to inquire. Perhaps she didn't know her exact age since she was illiterate. Maryam first came here when it was overrun by men.

Although she was an opium smoker, she managed to overdose on occasion. Once when she overdosed in a doorway, a passer-by thought she was deceased and dropped money next to her as *Zakat* or alms. After coming to, she was amazed to discover 100,000 Rials (USD4) beside her. Along with her brother, she resided with several peers. Interestingly, she passed her day with about 20 others. It sounded like she frequented a shooting gallery where heroin was bought and consumed on the premises. Yazd was her hometown, where she grew up with two brothers and two sisters. Although she commenced high school and enjoyed it, she dropped out after the second year. A few years later she picked up a job in a hospital and then married at 19. She led a quiet life, no alcohol or drugs, no trouble. Then when she was 26 something happened to her, which led her to use opium. The misfortune was not elaborated on and when asked about it, she just shrugged her shoulders and provided no more clues. Most of her life was spent being a housewife, supported by her husband without her own income, raising a couple of kids.

After using opium for 18 years, she graduated to smoking heroin. After three years of that, she was in trouble. 'I've been inside two, no, three times and every time it was because of these stupid drugs and what they have made me do. My last stint was for six months.'

In 25 years of drug-taking she'd abstained for just 36 days. So she must have used drugs in prison. Maryam's sense of compulsion to use had overshadowed all other things of pleasure or interest. By her own account, even though she experienced psychological and physical harm, her drug use continued, unabated. What's more she had carried on like this for two and a half decades.

When people develop a drug problem they usually fall foul of the law, as they often resort to crime to raise money to buy drugs. The crimes committed by our sample included drug dealing, fraud, crimes against property and violence. Maryam reminded me of the elderly woman I met at Evin Prison, the one who had already served several sentences. She told us that prisoners fashioned makeshift syringes out of an eye dropper and a pen. They took the soft rubber bulb off the dropper and connected it to the sheaf of a ballpoint pen to act as a syringe, though they still required a needle to puncture the skin to allow drugs to enter.

Some of our clients had been imprisoned at some time. Their main offence was property offences followed by drug possession and dealing. Many female prisoners had used heroin, even inside prison. But nowhere near as many as in the men's prison. It was difficult to determine the numbers involved, the number we might have to cater for. Somewhere from 10 to 50 out of every 100 females in prison might have used drugs. Such a wide range showed the difficulty in quantifying this behaviour. However, their consumption of drugs by injection was thought to be rare by women inside the big house.

As I left that day, I bumped into the clinic helper. He was obviously a user and by my reckoning on a dose of methadone that was too high, as he sweated profusely. He was a lanky dude, who wore his cap backwards and sucked at his teeth. He climbed the stairs four at a time up and down. He was a beanpole full of amphetamines. After I gave him a key ring earlier in the week, I couldn't shake him off my tail. He was opening doors, sweeping not so imaginary dirt with an imaginary broom. He took me to hail a taxi and told the driver in no uncertain terms to look after me; in fact, he swept away a few drivers with his imaginary broom before he settled on one that he could trust to drive me back to my hotel. My natural inclination is to jump in the front seat with the driver as we do back home, and also as there was a seat belt there but not in the back. My sweeper friend disapproved and kept holding the back door open for me, but I just waved him goodbye from the front seat. Most drivers don't like it, but I hopped in anyway and fished out the address card for my hotel.

*

On my return to Sydney, my first yearning was to swim in the ocean. During this time, I lived near Bondi Beach and would race down there at every opportunity. I had left a snowy Tehran and came back to an Australian mid-summer sizzling day. As my car turned from Bondi Road into Campbell Parade, the yellow crescent of the beach, speckled with people in colourful swimmers looked like a slice of fairy bread, white bread smothered in butter and sprinkled with hundreds and thousands—a sugary staple at any child's birthday party. Walking onto the beach was slightly jarring as most people were wearing swimmers or exercise gear and showing so much flesh, which contrasted sharply from the covered-up nation I had just left.

Chapter 7. Working with the Team

A request to deliver more training in Iran afforded me with another chance to visit, my third such one. I was keen to follow up with some of the clients I had met on my last visit and to observe the team at the clinic.

The two nurses worked five hours a day, six days a week. Their duties were to dispense methadone, distribute needles and syringes, provide condoms, change dressings and counsel and test for HIV. These positions were extremely troublesome to fill; we even had to suffice with other staff standing in to dispense methadone, which was not ideal for any length of time. Within a few months, though, two nurses were recruited who alternated duties between themselves. Usually, methadone was dispensed in a syrup form, but when the syrup was unavailable, physeptone tablets had to be crushed for clients to swallow.

One nurse, Parastoo, had graduated from nursing 24 years ago and worked on a psychiatric ward in a hospital. Unfortunately, Parastoo had polio as a child and ended up with a shorter leg and a limp. She was contemplating having an operation to lengthen her leg. This involved breaking the bone in her short leg and then placing pins into the bone above and below the cut. A metal device connected to the pins would be turned slowly, like a Chinese torture rack, to create a gap between the bones that keeps filling with new bone to produce an extension in the leg.

Although Parastoo was familiar with drug users, she had no experience with methadone treatment. Seyah observed her dispensing methadone to clients and was confident that Parastoo was competent in her role. Roya, the second nurse to join the team, had worked in a psychiatric unit. She preferred to distribute the harm reduction package. These little packages comprised two syringes, four needles, two condoms, a small container of sterile water and a plaster, all wrapped up several sheets of newspaper.

Roya thought that just a few clients were injecting and most were collecting harm reduction kits for their husbands, brothers or sons. Even though condoms were offered, very few were collected. Roya ran training courses for the clients on HIV and Hepatitis C, which she would repeat for new clients. She conducted HIV and Hepatitis

C testing. All the test results came back negative for HIV but 15 had Hepatitis C infection. They weren't injecting so perhaps they got it from tattooing. Or perhaps they were mistaken about whether they had injected! Actually, there was a lot of debate about how easy it was to transmit Hepatitis C via sex. Roya requested information about sexually transmissible Hepatitis C infection. It was frustrating that the nurses had received a work contract for just three months when it took so long to find them. Roya would often say it took many meetings to gain each woman's trust.

Laleh, the social worker, was responsible for case management and assisting with securing housing, employment and welfare entitlements. Laleh's role was to solve problems; she counselled them, trained them to make paper flowers to sell and taught other skills to enable some home cottage activities. Against good practice, Laleh called on clients at home and explored ways to improve their homes such as buying a carpet. Her involvement in the field of addiction covered four years, making her the most experienced and, a mentor to the others.

A few days later Zahra reappeared for an appointment with our doctor. Her shiny hair was dull and her white flowing dress soiled and crumpled. Her demure was despondent and she seemed frustrated. The interpreter and I pounced on her in a frantic attempt to cajole her into our line of thinking. Our new tact was a private meeting with Zahra in the director's office to elevate the status of our gathering. Over and over we hammered in the risks of dropping out of methadone, how it might affect the baby, how she might turn to drugs again. She looked sheepish at this point, as it appeared she was using drugs on top of her methadone or maybe, instead of that, selling her methadone to buy heroin. This would mean she was most likely injecting heroin, as she did before, possibly in a group setting and perhaps sharing syringes.

If we could transfer her to another centre closer to home would that help her to stay in treatment? No, it wouldn't. Round and round in circles we went.

Finally, thinking there must be something that would keep her here and safe, I put it to her 'What would keep you in treatment?'

'Nothing would,' she stated. She was determined to leave methadone and us behind.

Yesterday had been a busy day for the social worker having attended to 35 different clients. Fariba, a new client, was guided through the registration process, introduced to the services on offer and briefed about them by the staff. It would be Laleh who first asked clients about their drug use problems and family situation. She explored ways to refer them to other services such as Welfare Organization centres. She was responsible for vocational therapy and organized skill sharing among the clients in areas like sewing and making artificial flowers. She also coordinated client appointments with staff and coordinated staff meetings and training sessions. Training topics included life skills, identifying high risk situations, coping skills, and family problems. She discussed problems with clients in the safe room and was very busy, too busy. Initially she was too busy to meet me, sending a message informing me that we couldn't meet. I sent a message back to her, down the corridor, that I was ready to meet her, now. She was uncomfortable in our meeting, shifting in her seat. She requested more training, having already completed a course on counselling and individual and group therapy. She said one client wanted to divorce her husband, but she spoke to the husband and taught the client how to cook and dress and the client changed her mind about divorcing him. Divorcees faced a lot of stigma in Iran, she explained.

Fariba's matted hair poked out of her green hejab and fringed her pimply face. She wore a trench coat as her *Roopoosh*, tied tightly around her thin frame. She pushed her hands in her pockets and fiddled with a couple of keys inside. Her scarred face depicted the tough hand life had dealt her, which was at odds with her assertion that life was superb for her now. A small child clung to her leg and occasionally darted off to a corner in the room. In the focus group, her incessant babbling suggested she was intoxicated with a stimulant, probably methamphetamines. The cost of various drugs and ease of procurement were key indicators of any drug scene.

Fariba volunteered 'If you know a dealer you can score heroin quickly; otherwise it takes hours. It costs just a dollar or two for a hit.' She added 'that was five years ago, when I was using. When I was in prison, I didn't use drugs there. Drugs were too pricey; four, five times as much as they here on the street outside.'

She pointed a thumb over her shoulder at the open window and continued. 'And you better stash your drugs away or you have to divvy them up.' (Syringes were worth USD4 each inside, even worn out old bloody ones.) 'You know what?' she posed a rhetorical question to all present, 'they even use eye droppers as syringes; the inmates do. They sharpen the needle on the brick wall.' Her story about the drug scene in prison was very close to others' accounts.

As far back as Fariba's memory stretched her parents used *shriek*, an opium residue, just socially. But when Fariba was 12 and her brother died from leukemia, their use escalated. She lived in Tehran with her parents and three siblings. Her father was unfit to work so her mum cleaned houses. Before her mum shuffled off to work each day, she gave Fariba some opium as a baby to keep her placid. After a year or two her mum stopped giving opium to Fariba, but Fariba witnessed others using it. Eventually, she grew to hate drugs, and opium, in particular. 'I hassled them to quit, all the time.'

Her parents' preoccupation with opium meant the kids were left alone most days and nights. She ended up living with a brother. 'My brother's wife pushed her own ID card into my hand and instructed me to go and find a husband. "We can't support you," she said.'

While wandering the streets in Tehran, Fariba met her future husband. She was begging and sleeping rough in parks and sometimes her boyfriend gave her some money. Her boyfriend was from Kermanshah in the North West of Iran. Her boyfriend's father was a martyr who died during the war with Iraq.

She married at 17 years old, just before she had her first baby. Then she landed a job in a hospital doing errands for a few years. At 23 she suffered a migraine, so her husband gave her opium but told her it was codeine.

One of our key areas of concern for her was the duration of drug use she had endured before seeking help. For Fariba this had been a solid decade. They occasionally lived with his mother and both secretly used heroin daily. According to Fariba they paid USD8 a day to have two or three hits each.

On Fariba's first visit, she was unable to communicate without swearing. She had trust for no one and was angry—very angry and aggressive. Her life skills were non-existent. The social worker coaxed her back into behaving like a social being. Fariba was damaged from years of street living, knew nothing about cooking or cleaning and her personal hygiene was poor. So the staff taught her and helped her with her five-year-old daughter every visit. She left her husband and remarried.

Her second husband was 55 years old, though, and began opium use when he was 15. He supported her in treatment. Fariba's husband sought help elsewhere, and although he was rather unwell, he managed to work a day or two a week. Their baby, Avat, the little girl who accompanied her, was born an addict. I realised that she was always sleeping because Fariba was dosing her up on drugs! That was the same thing that had happened to her. Except her mother used opium while Fariba gave Avat methadone, we suspected. I asked the nurses to investigate.

During this trip, the person I was most concerned about was Mona. How Mona had fared over the last few months weighed on my mind. I half expected she had left treatment or even worse, had died. She was incredibly depressed, rocking back and forth in a chair. Her depression was severe. It had been almost a year since we last met. An appointment was arranged, and we met Mona one windy and wet afternoon. Immediately she denied any recent involvement in crimes or drugs, which were signals that she was on her way to recovering from drugs. But often methadone patients turn to stimulants like amphetamines when opiates failed to provide a buzz. Did this trap await her? Mona was becoming confident again and soon she was ready to take on some activity, even a craft class. It could be the first step in returning to work. We had two more important assessments; to investigate whether she had acquired HIV or Hepatitis C infection and whether she had traces of drugs in her urine. She willingly submitted to a blood test with the prerequisite counselling and to provide a urine sample.

Mona was still free of HIV infection for a second time. Unfortunately, she had acquired Hepatitis C infection, but when was unknown as she shunned the first test we offered. Perhaps she knew she had it then? The nurse counselled her when they tested her. The counselling session covered ways it could be passed to another, available treatments and where to receive treatment and how the disease might progress in Mona's case. More good news came from her urine test, which was clear of all drugs.

'It has been 220 days since I last used heroin,' boasted Mona.

Another area to investigate in order to build a complete picture of her health and where she was in her recovery included social functioning. Her appearance had blossomed, according to the lawyer. Her makeup was being removed and freshly applied on a daily basis. Her clothes were looking smart and she was smiling, laughing even. Mona's days evolved into a stable routine, with her retiring early in the evening and eating regular meals. No longer were her days preoccupied with some scam to raise money, to buy drugs and then to find somewhere to use them. Withdrawals, which plagued her, were over. The staff had influenced her routine somewhat, by insisting she fronted up at a certain time to collect her methadone. As long as she stayed with us, she had a fair chance of improving. How long she needed to stay was unknown, but probably years.

Over a cup of tea Mona confessed to having slipped up last month. But the time before that was months ago. An assessment of her drug use found she was not preoccupied by drugs anymore. The last time we spoke she was in a temporary marriage, which was still the case. Mona and her husband were sexually active and always used condoms. She proudly stated it was a year since she had sex when she was high on drugs. When someone was high, they were more likely to put themselves at risk of HIV, other infections or an unwanted pregnancy. And her two friends had come back into her life, providing some support for her, calling on her often and socialising with her. No longer did she hang out with users. These aspects of how Mona spent her day indicated she was improving. Now that she was off heroin, she felt many aches and pains, ones she was unaccustomed to.

But had her mood responded to treatment, I wondered? Previously Mona had been severely depressed, suicidal, rocking back and forth in her chair. From her appearance her mood seemed to have lifted. Another assessment of her mental state revealed that her mood had indeed lifted from being severely depressed to being moderately depressed.

Mona summed up her mood, 'I don't feel so grumpy. I've cut down on my smoking. I have just six cigarettes a day now, not one after the other.'

Cutting down on smoking would not have saved much money, as cigarettes were dirt cheap. So it was unlikely that money was the reason for her cutting back. But since cigarettes were the last thing that people clung to, it was suggestive of another hill climbed on her road to recovery. On she went listing more areas of improvement; never missing methadone, showering daily and not having a drug problem now. I wanted to believe her but struggled to do so.

Mona still lived in her own house and had picked up some odd jobs. Meanwhile her husband earned money by ferrying passengers on his motorbike. Apparently, there was no conflict with her family or friends. Mona was eager to share stories about her life before drugs, when she had achieved many goals. What would help her return to work? Money, Mona said. A lack of it was her major problem. She required money to divorce her husband, to secure her own flat and visit her daughter.

I made a point of asking the lawyer about her case one more time. The reason for hiring a lawyer was to aid with legal matters. I raised the issue with the director, showing him the staff descriptions and read it to him. He didn't respond to that but had already decided not to fill the lawyer's position once she left.

The director then shared his impressions of the service; previously he had some very serious misgivings about working with female drug users. According to him, it was unheard of to help sex workers in Iran. How would others respond? Indeed, in the early days there was a firebomb threat because it was rumoured that the clinic was a brothel. Swift action was required to avert the attack. Then a female pimp came to the service to see if she could recruit sex workers for her brothel.

On he went. Workers were freezing in winter when moving from one room to another along the external corridor and the rooms themselves were icy. As funding was tight how could they heat the rooms in an economical way?

The administrator had the good fortunate to participate in a workshop on drugs in Europe, which enlightened her. On her return she announced to everyone that the main issue was the law; drugs were illegal. Also, she managed to inspect some services and compare how those services operated in relation to her service. There was an obligation to pay superannuation for staff, but she had discovered one scheme that offered a discount of paying 10% instead of 30%. It was unclear if this meant the staff would receive less super than the required amount. Another Iranian agency involved in our project had a similar problem with the payment of superannuation.

Many of our free services were unavailable elsewhere or were very expensive, such as those delivered by the midwife and the lawyer. The main clinic had over 500 male clients until a new law came into force limiting the caseload to 200. Still, it was rather daunting space to be in, especially if you were a woman.

Then it was my turn to raise a few complaints with the director. When one client broke her leg, she was unable to collect her methadone and was denied any take-home doses. She had to go through withdrawal from methadone, which was horrible. Methadone withdrawal can be very uncomfortable. Symptoms include nausea, vomiting, fever, chills and aches and pains in the joints. Some people can even feel suicidal, depressed, tired and experience hallucinations and panic attacks. She then had to recommence on methadone. Disappointingly, the director thought this problem rested with the client rather than the doctor. It was essential to solve these problems. The policy was that clients were prohibited from having take-home doses but surely there could have been some arrangement made for this woman. Perhaps she could have been assisted to reach us to receive a reducing dose for a week so as to avoid severe withdrawals. Other complaints were about the opening hours and clients having their dose reduced if they missed three doses in a row. While this seemed harsh, it was actually a safety measure as their tolerance for the drug would have waned.

With the staff settling into a routine, the ups and down of working there began to tell on the staff. The psychologist, for example, said her group therapy sessions on drug cravings, life skills and parenting were suffering from a high turnover of participants. I was unconvinced of the usefulness of such group therapy sessions. Usually, these clients were so damaged that they were unable to function appropriately in such sessions. The rules that participants in therapy had to follow were often beyond these people. For example, confidentiality was a crucial rule that was applied without exception, yet many were unable to appreciate how one must keep another's confidence. The types of misdemeanours one confessed to in a group therapy session were fodder for these busy bodies; crimes that have gone unpunished, scams to obtain money and drugs and even continued drug use while in therapy. Also, group therapy required participants to have empathy for each other. Part of my role was to assist the workers but also to allow them to discover their own way of dealing with the issues. So I queried the utility of these groups but didn't urge them to stop. Then the psychologist held group discussions on the harms of substance abuse, and the reason why clients sought treatment. Nine clients turned up to blame their husbands for their problems and heroin for the reason for seeking treatment. As a result, the psychologist was approached to provide individual counselling. It took some time to find the right balance between group therapy versus individual therapy.

The social worker's initial efforts at employment training floundered. Two enthusiastic souls were trained in textile and bag making to assist her to run a class, yet they were warring with their husbands and could only attend intermittently. Often, they turned up, ate breakfast, smoked a few cigarettes in the safe room and then left for the day. While it might appear therapeutic to provide jobs, most were unlikely to perform at the required level—they were in medical treatment for a serious addiction. I questioned the wisdom of giving them so much responsibility so soon.

Another class was making artificial flowers to be sold at the markets, earning the makers some pocket money. One class covered life skills and how to identify high risk situations where one might be tempted to revert to drugs. The social worker also taught coping skills; ways of dealing with family problems. She would position herself in the safe room and hold fort with whoever came in. For our folk, the basics of life can be insurmountable; assisting them into a daily routine was a challenge. When they first came along, at least half were staying up all night, taking drugs, having sex or doing whatever. But attendance at our service required clients to present every day between 8 am and 3 pm; otherwise, their dose of methadone was forfeited.

The social worker was available six days a week and even called on clients at home to assess their financial and social situation, after which she might refer them to a welfare centre. I felt decidedly uncomfortable about her venturing out to their homes and urged her to reconsider, or at least let another accompany her. After about six months, the social worker became fed up and stopped helping the research assistants and began shouting at clients. It sounded like she had burnt out.

The lawyer was about to resign. Most of the legal hassles concerned clients' husbands, like getting a divorce. But a divorce was probably not the best option for most women as they were dependent on their husbands in many ways, not just financially. Other common legal matters included applying to foster a child, obtaining a National ID card, escaping domestic violence and financial problems, such as cashing a cheque or claiming an inheritance. She also had a number of custody battles on her books. Although the lawyer was only available one day a week, clients lined up for legal aid.

The free meals had stopped, although they began again two days before my visit, but it was just a watery soup. With funds dwindling, meals were the first item to be cut. There seemed to be a range of complaints, mostly minor ones. So I asked whether they knew there was another clinic for them to attend. Some said they didn't know about it, though I doubted that as such information would spread quickly among clients. Some said that the clients at the other clinic were different. They dealt drugs and some were homeless. It seemed a little odd to me that they had no hesitation in displaying their prejudice, but I guessed the stigma attached to some of these attributes prevailed here as well.

The doctor's cousin was a dentist with links to a dental university. The doctor arranged for clients to be treated by dental students for a fraction of the standard cost. As many clients had serious dental problem, we assumed that, even though the university was miles away, the reduced fee was incentive enough to get one's teeth fixed. However, no one went to the dental university.

The safe room was in the middle of the building and like all the other rooms, opened onto the corridor. Some rooms, the ones the psychologist and the social worker used, had been painted. The furniture in the safe room was moved aside waiting for the painters, including a large table that usually sat in the middle of the room. Oddly though, the clients preferred the room with the large table, which enabled them to spread out their possessions like a shopkeeper and her wares. I had insisted a room be set aside where women could chat and drink tea and just be. The room also provided a focal point for staff to engage with them in a relaxed environment. The room was their sanctuary where hejabs could be removed and cigarettes smoked.

One day two clients sat in the room, talking but not smoking, which was unusual as virtually every drug user smoked and quite heavily. One lady had a brochure on Hepatitis C and read out the symptoms to her friend who was fossicking through her bag.

She asked, 'fever? Do you have a fever?'

'No,' the friend answered.

On the first woman went, 'fatigue?'

'Yes, I'm always tired' was the reply.

'Vomiting? Have you vomited lately?' she asked her friend.

'No,' she shook her head, before asking 'do I have hepatitis?'

'Yeah. Maybe... no... I don't know,' her friend said.

When I asked if they had any complaints, both clients said they were happy with the staff. Neither had any suggestions for how we could improve the place.

They had shut the door for privacy, but the paint fumes were still overwhelming. I had to open the door. The coordinator was with me to interpret and there were five clients plus one child. This was about the third time I had seen that child and I wondered how often she attended school. She seemed like a lovely kid. Raising kids was a trial enough without the added burden of a drug habit to preoccupy you. The psychologist told me she ran a parenting course. Hopefully the cycle of an addicted parent having a child who develops a habit later in life could be broken.

It was time for another focus group. The next topic we quizzed them about was their sex lives. Most of the interrogation occurred during their first few visits, so it was encouraging that they were willing to open up to us so early on. The area of sexual activity was left a little longer, though. About half told us they had a partner, and a few admitted to having several partners, concurrently. People who use drugs tend to neglect their health including their sexual health. Our midwife conducted Pap smear tests and half had a mild inflammation, but one woman had severe inflammation. No cases of warts or herpes were found, but two cases of fungi were noted and all tests for syphilis were negative.

Then we moved on to the topic of prison. Almost half of our group had been incarcerated, which indicated that we were reaching a risky group, the one that had prompted us to set up the service. While some admitted using drugs in the big house, none reported injecting them. Nor did anyone report any sex inside the prison walls.

Painting the walls had not made the place any prettier than before; it was still ugly. Nevertheless, the clients often mentioned that they liked the atmosphere, so maybe we were too fussy about its presentation. But the building had its own problems. The electricity kept cutting out and the computers were often going down, preventing the administrator from sending regular reports on the activities some weeks.

The coordinator, the doctor, the midwife and the administrator met to discuss these and other problems. They decided to buy some common medications such as antibiotics, vaginal creams and ointments. Also, the administrator made an agreement with a nearby pharmacy and laboratory for referral when necessary. All agreed that these services should not be advertised widely among the clients or they would pressure the staff to do unnecessary procedures just because they were free. The coordinator wondered if we have a similar problem in Australia, people availing themselves to services just because they were free. She said this was common in Iran. It would take some time to establish a good network of referrals as there was likely to be some resistance from other agencies to provide services to our people, but we hoped with time that these agencies would relent.

When the director decided to split the opening hours so the women could come in the morning and the men in the afternoon, it took some time for a few men to register the new time. Those male clients who couldn't remember the new time were very dishevelled in tatty clothes and underweight. Their look was one of desperation. Their weight loss could have been due to drug use or perhaps to being HIV positive. Whatever the reason, women were reluctant to be near these male users. This timeshare arrangement saved money on the rent for the premises and expensive items like a safe in which to store methadone.

After Roya, one of nurses, broke her arm, her role of HIV and Hepatitis C testing was neglected. Testing clients for HIV infection was important for them and for us as we had a particular interest in whether we were preventing HIV and Hepatitis C transmission. Tests were scheduled for certain dates and missing some tests would hamper the research. In a matter of weeks, Roya was back taking blood samples and counselling about ways to avoid HIV infection. The case load of clients had reached 40, but as soon as we had gathered up some new clients, others had scampered back to the streets of South Tehran. This turnover of clients happened early in their time with us, usually in the first three days. If we didn't interview and test soon after their arrival, we would miss recruiting them at this point. So if we recruited a woman who then left, we would most likely catch her on the next round. Then we could resume the treatment and the research once more, rather than starting afresh.

Possible reasons for leaving treatment early were considered. Perhaps the dose of methadone they started on with was inadequate. Or was the rate of increase in the dose of methadone unsatisfactory? The nurses monitored patients very closely looking for possible explanations. It should be easy to rectify if this dosage was indeed the case. No one had studied females who smoked heroin, so we had to calculate the dose of methadone with some trial and error. The researcher decided to interview clients who were friends of those who had left. I left Iran wondering when I would be able to visit again.

*

Not long after I returned home, I was awoken from a deep sleep one night when my phone rang. A foreign voice shouted down the line. 'No one takes the condoms, what do we do?'

At first, I was unsure who was calling, and then I recognised her accent. It was the administrator. I couldn't work out how she had my number.

'OK, OK,' I said dozily, 'put them on the front counter so they don't have to ask for them. Let them take some without being seen.'

Click. She hung up immediately and presumably moved the said items up front for everyone to help themselves. Up until then, only a measly 20 condoms a month were being collected, not enough to upset a pope. This number rose to 100 in November and reached 400 by February. By the year's end, we were distributing almost a thousand condoms a month (Dolan et al., 2011a). Even if they were passing them onto others, we didn't mind as others were protecting themselves, their partners or others in their circle of friends. It was the same pattern with syringes. They had collected syringes, but, by all accounts, they weren't injecting. I asked the staff to quiz them about this. Apparently, some clients grabbed syringes for relatives who were injecting. One lady told us that her husband and all three sons were on the needle. That has got to be a disaster waiting to happen, if it hadn't already happened. This gang would need to be dismantled, if anyone was to recover from drugs.

Chapter 8. The Money-go-round

From the outset, I revelled in the challenge of securing funding for our venture. When Bijan and I concocted our plan for the service, approaching funders was our priority. We approached numerous potential funders without success for some time. I sent a grant proposal to the Bill Gates' Global Fund charity but got knocked back. Over the next three years, I submitted over a dozen funding requests, almost one every three months. Every single one was turned down. I fired off proposals to America, to the UK, the Middle East, to Europe and to Australia. Slowly I came to realise I might never find any funder for this project.

After each rejection, we refined the proposal, making it more ambitious, perhaps too ambitious. Targeting American funders was probably not the best source of funding for a project based in the Islamic Republic of Iran, although it was worth targeting international organisations based in the US. Initially the project had aimed to treat women in prison, like those wretched souls I had encountered in Evin Prison, who would then be transferred to our clinic once released. This approach might just sever the pattern of being repeatedly jailed and released. How we would secure funding for a project that included all the components we were proposing—a prison methadone program, a community-based centre and a rather complicated program of research—had seemed doubtful.

The coordinator received a call from the prison saying they were ready to begin and had a dozen or so women who could benefit from treatment. As they seemed willing, it was time to train prison staff in assessing clients. We thought we could count on their support for the project, but the departure of our main contact at prison meant that we had to negotiate a new agreement to continue. This issue became a serious concern for our funder. The new prison director rang our coordinator to say she knew nothing of this project. She could not find any documentation on file. She requested a formal letter introducing the project, but we were not to mention the previous dealings we had with the prison department. The coordinator asked us to solve this problem; otherwise, she doubted whether we could continue. The prison people had a few problems with the proposal and called for more information. The coordinator sent more information but the problems they were highlighting couldn't be solved by providing more information. Consequently, the funder contemplated delaying the second instalment until these issues were resolved. Furthermore, as there was some uncertainty about how the first instalment would be used, if the prison component was abandoned. The overall project might have to cease.

We came to realise the prison part of the project had to be excluded. Key prison players were unable to write a letter indicating that they were withdrawing from the project because it would show a disability on their part. Yet my university required this letter to cancel the contract. I felt trapped.

The independent accountant made everyone feel just that bit more at ease about how the funding was to be spent. This fellow would send financial reports to Australia on a monthly basis. The reports were presented in three fluorescence colours with all expenditure listed in Iranian Rials and US and Australian dollars.

We managed to wire the first instalment without trouble to the research centre, the clinic and to the prison NGO. When the second funding instalment appeared in our university bank account, I thought the funding hassles were essentially over. I had not, of course, reckoned on sanctions on fund transfers to Iran being wound up a notch. By the time the second instalment of funds was due to be disbursed, the UN had increased sanctions against Iran. During our project the UN imposed three sets of sanctions against Iran; in December 2006, in March 2007 and then in March 2008. Broadly, the sanctions were related to uranium enrichment and nuclear weapons. So in theory the transfer of funds to Iran for public health purposes should have been permitted.

Having the money in Sydney was futile if we couldn't transfer it. Unless we could transfer the second instalment to Iran, the clinic would have to close, and the service would stop. Attempts to transfer funds via our university bank were blocked. A protracted discussion occurred about this for months. We battled with our university finance department, which seemed reluctant to transfer the funds. Our bank responded with ten questions requiring explanation for the funds transfer. Even though sufficient justification was furnished, the bank seemed unwilling or unable to transfer the funds. For five months our finance person and I tried to overcome the bank's adherence to the sanctions. I was confident the money would be used for the intended purpose as our Iranian accountant was in charge of distributing the money to the three groups. The sanctions were proving to be insurmountable. I asked the finance section at my university if they would issue a bank cheque that could be cashed in Iran. But there was no way to cash an overseas bank cheque in Iran. The research centre was due another payment, which was slowing their ability to deliver which was impacting on our obligations to the funder. It was necessary to find another way to transfer the funds. As our researcher had moved to Europe, she thought she may be able to forward the funds from there, so we transferred the money to her. But as soon as the money landed in her account the bank took a commission of EU€400, even though they were unable to move the money to Iran. The bank manager told her it was due to the sanctions against Iran. After several weeks she was asked to return the funds since they could not go via Italy. It must have been tempting to receive a large amount of money deposited into your bank account while you were in a foreign country. But I knew the researcher would return the money, in its entirety and without delay.

Meanwhile our actual budget didn't tally with the proposal's budget. This discrepancy had to be rectified, immediately. This financial irregularity would worry the funder. Thankfully, the funder was unconcerned that the project was falling behind schedule. But the delay would have a knock-on effect for future reporting and milestones. They wanted to amend our contract in light of the delays and the changed circumstances with the prison component.

Another avenue to explore was to use a money exchange centre in Iran that had an account in Australia from where we could send the funds. It was necessary to find a centre that we could trust, but how would you know? I had heard of small convenience stores in North Sydney that could transfer money to Iran, but again how would you know they were reliable? What recourse would you have if the money disappeared? Another option was to transfer the funds through the World Health Organization (WHO). A man from the WHO thought it possible, but a contract would have to be drawn up with the WHO collecting a commission of 13%. The problem was it could be weeks before such a contract would be signed and then some more time to wire the funds. In 2012, another request to deliver training gave me the opportunity to visit Iran once more.

One option was for a traveller to Iran to carry cash on their person; AUD60,000. As I was travelling there soon, there was an expectation I would carry the money. I would have felt like a drug runner carrying that much money. It just sounded too risky, even for me to consider. Then Persepolis ran out of funding for salaries. Next month they wouldn't be able to pay for methadone. I dreaded the thought of 40 or so people being forced off methadone, back on the streets and back on heroin or opium in a day or two.

Meanwhile, another attempt to transfer the money was made. One bank suggested using British sterling as that had worked in the past. We were desperate. Once more, I had to answer questions relating to the transfer. The director rang to say he would be closing the doors at the end of the month, in eight days' time, if no funds were forthcoming. Then a check with the bank revealed the funds had left our account, €32,000 had been transferred yesterday! But while it had left our account, it had yet to reach Iran, where it was a holiday to celebrate the nationalisation of the oil industry. I received an urgent call from the bank. Again, we were interrogated as to the reason for wanting to transfer funds to Iran. 'What was the economic purpose of this transaction? What was the nature of goods or services concerned and when was this agreement made?' I repeated the answers that I had already given twice. I prayed the money would appear in our colleagues' bank accounts this time. Once the research centre received theirs, we assumed the clinic had, too. But it hadn't. At least I could placate the director that the funds were coming, as some of it had reached another organisation in Tehran.

Initially, we were not allowed to have a contract with the Iranian Prison Department, nor were we able to transfer funds directly to them, so an NGO filled this intermediary role. However, once the prison component was cancelled, we had to cancel our contract with the NGO and request they return the first payment. I politely requested the NGO to transfer their unspent funds to the clinic, rather than return them to us. The coordinator and the accountant had not been paid this month, or last month. I was pleasantly relieved to hear the NGO transferred their funds to the clinic, but this was just a temporary measure. Of course, as the project had commenced months ago, the expenses were building up. They were desperate for the entire amount of money to be transferred. The accountant recommended a bank in Germany. Bijan suggested the Bank of Tehran as they did business with banks in France, UK, Germany and Finland. But none of these suggestions worked.

Finally, I pleaded with the funder to send the funds directly from their office to Iran. Somehow a Swiss charity might have a better possibility of success. They duly instructed their bank in Switzerland to send the funds to Iran via Germany. They were informed that their accounts had been debited so we had assumed the funds were making their way to Iran.

But the funds that were still sitting in Australia had to be transferred to Iran. Then our accountant mentioned his company had an account in a Dubai bank and that we could use that. Finally, the funds were transferred from Switzerland to Dubai to Germany and to Iran. This allowed us and the researchers to continue their work. And no one was forced off the program, though some staff wages were delayed for a month or two.

While visiting our service was my prime aim, I was also requested to run a training course for about 40 prison doctors from all over Iran, focusing on drug withdrawal and treatment. It was snowing that day—another example of Iran's confounding stereotypes in my mind. The training was geared towards prison doctors but covered topics relevant for drug workers, so I asked if our staff and those from another service could attend.

I did wonder if I could skip the training, but I would have let down my colleague and all the doctors who had travelled from all over the country to Tehran. One guy who had turned up at this training had been at my first training some six years earlier. I was happy to meet him again. After that first training, he accompanied us to his prison in Shiraz.

One training activity required participants to list the characteristics of prisons and prisoners. Surprisingly every suggestion from the participants was relevant to prisons and prisoners in Australia. Although I had the pleasure of visiting many prisons in Iran, I still thought perhaps the other ones might be different. This activity reassured me that the conditions were similar between our countries and within this one. More importantly it meant that programs that worked for prisoners in one country, such as drug treatment and HIV prevention, would most likely work for prisoners in other countries. Topics included how to assess if an inmate had a drug problem, how to treat these problems and human rights for prisoners. And we discussed how many government elections had a law-and-order platform, which usually meant punitive approaches towards criminals rather than rehabilitative ones. Prisons were a no-win story for governments as far as the media were concerned. If the government was doing something good, they were "too soft." If they were not doing enough, they were also criticised. This applied as much in Iran as in Australia or other Western countries.

I was training the frontline workers; the doctors and nurses who saw prisoners every day. Iran was more progressive than most countries in the West and the Middle East in how they tackled HIV in prison. I made a point of congratulating them on this. I was fairly certain that most wouldn't really have known what other countries were doing. So I outlined where Iran stood in the world in terms of addressing HIV in prisons. I had decided to cover treatments other than methadone as these doctors were already providing this form of treatment. In fact, in terms of methadone treatment coverage of prisoners, Iran ranked about tenth in the world and first among developing countries. This country was serious about preventing HIV and aiding people to recover from drug dependency. At the break, I met with the head of the prison organisation. We had a quick discussion and I suggested some areas for research and she told me they were already looking at these areas. When a country has such impressive programs, they need to be studied. There had been a major study of methadone in Iranian prisons but somehow it didn't quite work out. It appeared the way the study was carried out had a few problems with it. This was such a shame as there were so few randomised controlled trials of methadone programs for prisoners.

As the training came to a close, there was the customary exchange of gifts. I had made sure to bring a suitcase full of presents for whomever I met. Yet I was still to be outdone. The prison boss had two presents for me: a red coarse rug and a huge enamel plate. The rug was small, and the pattern was intricate, depicting an ancient story of the Persian Empire before Islam came to Iran. The enamel plate was large and blue with a scalloped edge, only to be brought out on special occasions. I had brought a dozen sterling silver cheese knives with a kangaroo on the handle and was pleased to be able to offer one to her. On a previous visit I had made the mistake of bringing ties for the guys, until Bijan told me that the strict Muslims shun ties because they symbolise the western world. I had brought a boomerang for one friend's young children and had practiced and practiced throwing it, but never got the chance to show off.

*

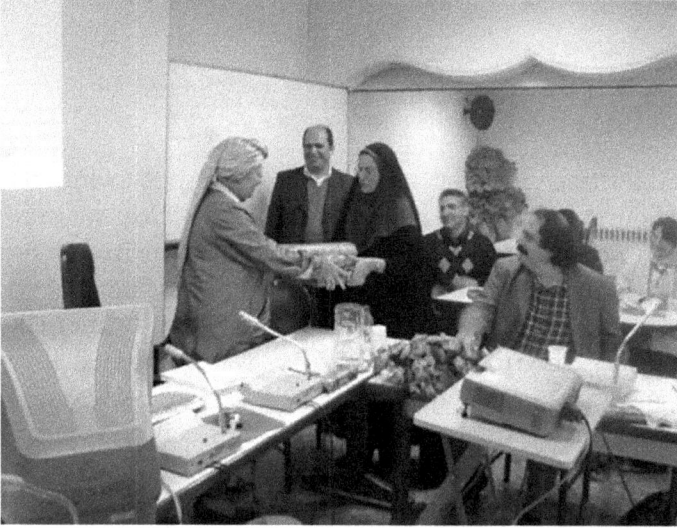

The author and the prison director exchange gifts

The workers were still pestering the director that they needed a psychiatrist and he was pestering me. I examined the budget to find if some item could be moved around. But they were after another USD8,000 for the psychiatrist and the promised winter kits. The kit was to contain a coat, socks, a scarf and gloves for the coming winter, especially for the homeless. I set about finding the extra money so they could be a little warmer through the winter and perhaps a bit more contented, if we could hire a psychiatrist.

Spring was on its way and the winter kits could wait until next year. Meanwhile the amended budget, which excluded the prison component, had been accepted by the funder. The research centre had wanted to buy some computers for goodness sake! Coming from a wealthy research centre, I just assumed they had spare computers sitting on a desk somewhere. But, as their budget was for salaries only and they required two computers, I had to explain we were unable to pay for additional expenses that were not in the contract.

Although we knew the prison component was cancelled, we received official notice in the report for the month of *Dey* (22nd of December to 20th of January). It simply said 'The prison project will not happen.' Meanwhile a methadone program had commenced for female prisoners in Iran. At least women were able to join our community program once released from prison. I left Iran feeling fairly satisfied with all that we were achieving.

Chapter 9. Life at the Clinic

While exhausting financial negotiations were occupying my time in Sydney, client numbers continued to grow. It was clear we were meeting a need and word had gotten around. I had been invited to present our results at Iran's National Drug Conference. During my fifth trip, I reviewed the clinic's progress and, more importantly, met clients once more. They sent my itinerary. Every day was accounted for with two or three meetings each day from the day I arrived. I was running a workshop for prison doctors, visiting another centre, visiting a rebirth shelter whatever that was and more meetings. I was told it was not possible to visit prison this time. I was determined to be at the clinic as much as I could. Also, I had to review my master's student's progress. She had evaluated another female-only drug service, so I was very keen to hear her research.

My first day back at the clinic saw a resumption of the focus groups that I so enjoyed on my previous trips. The coordinator wandered around asking if anyone had something to share. The topic was open today. She had one person in mind, if only she could find her. After a few trips up and down the stairs she found Fariba, both were beaming. I couldn't image what to expect. The group took shape around her. She sat centre stage, ready to deliver one of the most moving stories to date.

Fariba and her boyfriend travelled to Kermanshah a hot spot for drugs, although he was not using drugs at this time. Her family was unable to care for her, but when they hadn't heard from her for some time, they showed her photo to the police and asked for assistance in locating her. They police found her and brought her to the police station for a reprimand to teach her a lesson. Her mother and uncle came to the police station. The uncle beat her because she had run away, and he beat her boyfriend as well. He coerced her mother to consult a doctor to determine if she was still a virgin.

Fariba confessed that she had had sex with him but that was her first time. Tears welled up in her eyes as she revealed her painful past. 'Mum didn't tell me how to protect myself against any danger or threats and I knew zero about sex. My boyfriend professed his love and promised to marry me so that's why I had sex with him. My boyfriend and I were sent to juvenile detention. For the first two months we were just friends then we married, in the detention centre. I was 13. When we were released, we slept in parks but I didn't have sex with him. During the day he went to military service. I felt like an orphan. I had not a soul to confide in, to help with my problems. I never had the chance to attend school, I can't even write my name. In detention I suffered as I had no money to buy things, we were given just food. My parents didn't visit me. When we were released, he took me to Kermanshah where we lived together for two years.'

Her young daughter was tugging at her *Roopoosh*, wanting something or other. She seemed to respond to her in a caring way; maybe the harms of her parents' drug use had not trickled down to her daughter, Avat, or maybe it was because we were watching. The five-year-old girl was very lively, not quite ready for school. Perhaps next year, Fariba sighed.

Her puffy hands revealed many desperate attempts of shoving needles under the skin to find tiny spider-like veins. Her teeth were brown stumps from little brushing and much smoking. Her skin looked leathery, yet she was smiling all the time.

'My mother-in-law used to beat me up and make me do chores; cook, clean but I didn't know how to do those things. I was just 14 years old. She would beat me with a hose. But one day while I was being beaten, I hit back and escaped. My husband was still doing his military service during the days and returning home at weekends. So I divorced him. Actually, that's when my misery began.

'I went back to living on the streets. Afghan refugees who also lived on the streets, used to beat me up, but I could defend myself. They assaulted me physically, not sexually. I fought back, swearing and shouting and swinging my fists at them. Some street kids befriended me and introduced me to a woman who was a pimp. Although the pimp wasn't an addict, she gave me some bloody opium to do my job. I wasn't a sex worker; I cleaned her place in exchange for food and shelter. By my 17th birthday, I was injecting heroin. In winter, I slept in large garbage bins to keep warm. I reckon I went to prison every year I was on heroin. I smuggled drugs and went to prison for that. I stole some things and went to prison. I bashed someone and went to prison. I never used heroin inside, though, you know. Drugs were so expensive in there. But I told the guards, I will use heroin when I get out.'

'I'm 40 now so how long I have been sticking needles in myself? Well, I stopped using heroin three years ago when I came here. So how long was I trapped in that world of drugs and thugs? Nineteen terrible long years.'

She relayed more of her story. 'I was homeless, sleeping on the streets and in parks for years. I have been attacked many times. All my belongings have been stolen.' Her voice rose and she clenched her hands together as she spoke. 'I was left with just the clothes I wore. I slept under bridges to stay dry and went for days, weeks even, without showering. I took syringes out of bins and off the streets and used them without a second thought. I was lucky I didn't get AIDS. Then someone told me about this place, but at first I did not trust her. I couldn't believe that such a place would exist for someone like me.'

She turned to another woman and said 'You remember Fafa? She brought me here. Still I thought it may have been a trap. Why would they care about me when no one else had? I have turned my life around. I have gotten married and I have a young child. My husband doesn't use drugs. Our home is very small but it's ours and believe it or not I have given up drugs. I couldn't have done it on my own.'

I suspected she was right that she couldn't have turned her life around without the help of the staff and its services—well, not in such a short time. Her story really summed up the poor self-esteem that most had when they finally sought treatment. Most people give up drugs but usually it takes years, many years and then some to gain an inch of self-worth.

She heard that there was methadone in the female prison now so they would be happy. Another woman joked that it would be good to be on methadone in prison as you didn't have to travel like you do on the outside. Most lived some distance from we were located and found the trip inconvenient.

'I can try and fool myself but not my God,' Fariba said, holding her hands up in a surrender pose. 'I have used heroin since starting treatment,' she went on, bowing her head. 'But I haven't used heroin for three years. I had some crystal meth two months ago. Occasionally, I use opium with my husband—he is aggressive,' she added, as if to excuse her drug use. 'I have to cope with living with him, but it's better than sleeping on the streets. I was forced to have an abortion against my will; I wanted to keep it. I have a good rapport with my five stepchildren. My parents have passed away. I have no relationship with my brothers.'

Fariba ended with high praises for the staff. 'I am pleased with them and think they do their job really well.'

After having toughed it out on the streets, though, her benchmark of a good service was always going to be at the lower end of acceptability.

The waitress glided in with tea. Fariba picked up a sugar cube and placed it between her teeth and proceeded to suck her tea through the cube. The social worker motioned for us to move into another room for a private chat. There was more background to our young friend that the social worker felt compelled to brief us on.

Not only did she have to be re-socialized, but they also had to work with her husband. When Fariba became pregnant with Avat, her husband didn't know if he was the father. So, at first he refused to apply for a birth certificate. The staff convinced him over several sessions to take care of his child, to be responsible. Since then, he has bought a small apartment and has added his name to the birth certificate. He commenced saving money for the baby's future. Work continued with the husband as he complained that Fariba stayed out late. Their marriage was a temporary one. The social worker continued, telling us that Fariba had four children, from three different husbands. Three kids were raised in an orphanage but would be teenagers now. Perhaps the drug using harm had trickled down the line to her kids.

If Fariba was wary about coming here perhaps others were as well. Although we had a reasonable caseload, I felt we could accommodate more women. So I asked the group for their opinion on what would draw people to us. One young woman said 'No one knows about it; you got to advertise it.' Another raised her concerns about the reduced level of care they would receive if more users came along. 'If there are more patients coming here maybe I won't get to see the doctor when I want to.' Active drug users are not known for their generous side, at least not until they are in recovery. An older woman said that the mix of clients was good as we are all similar, but, at the other clinic, she nodded her head to one side, many of the clients are homeless. She went on to say, 'I'm glad they don't come here. I don't like being around homeless clients.'

I was dismayed by this as she had just heard Fariba's story and was announcing this in her presence. Another woman wanted the service to be opened for more hours.

An old problem had resurfaced. The staff had run out of methadone syrup again as sometimes it was difficult to import it. So Physeptone or methadone tablets had to be crushed up to be distributed to the clients. One of the clients was worried about reports on television that methadone causes cancer. Funny how they were all so worried about methadone causing cancer yet continued smoking, puffing away on cigarettes that they knew caused cancer and injecting drugs which were adulterated with who knew what. So the doctor agreed to hold a session about the myths of methadone and also to raise the issue of the harms of smoking cigarettes.

*

Soon Ramadan would be here. In preparation for the fast through the day, the cook prepared *sahari*, a meal which Muslims eat before dawn. *Adas-polo* was on the menu today, a delicious and hearty dish made of aromatic basmati rice, lentils, caramelized onion, raisins and spices and served with chicken. This meal would be served to those outside at 4 am! During Ramadan, Muslims must abstain from eating and drinking during daylight hours, so you can imagine quite a feast is served when dusk settles in. Conjugal relations between a husband and wife are forbidden during the daylight hours. Apart from adhering to the requirements of Ramadan, Muslims must acknowledge God and Muhammad as His Messenger, pray five times a day and pay *zakat*. Giving alms or *zakat*, is when the wealthy pay a set amount of their wealth to the poor. And Muslims should make the pilgrimage to Mecca, at least once in their life. One should try to curtail one's worldly pastimes as much as possible during Ramadan. By fasting one foregoes physical comfort, creating a sense of equality between the rich and poor.

As quite a number of clients were religious, staff organised a day trip to a religious site. On the birthday of the daughter of Mohammad the Prophet, there was a small celebration with some entertainment and gifts for the clients. Also, some religious clients felt uncomfortable discussing sex and, more importantly, safe sex. They felt these issues should not be discussed openly. The midwife modified her working style to minimise this discomfort and invited those likely to be offended in group discussions, for a private consultation.

Most days I positioned myself in the safe room, smoking cigarettes and drinking tea. Some clients were watching television and, when a show with traditional music came on, they began to laugh and clap their hands. The safe room felt lovely to be in. It had only been six years in the making. Two more women-only clinics had opened in Tehran, and one was in South Tehran, just like ours. Apparently, they offered similar services to ours so they might have an impact on our project. I urged our staff to meet the workers, so they could coordinate their efforts and perhaps have similar rules for clients, so they can enforce them across the board.

Today there were 39 patients registered. The doctor said there were four new clients last week, but some others had slipped away. One regular client left when her husband was released from prison and they got straight back into drugs. This was a recurring theme, one spouse leading the other astray. Most women had a partner who also used drugs and, in reality, if they wanted quit drugs, they had to quit relationships with drug users, or cajole their partners into care at the same time.

In the safe room, the large wooden boardroom table had been replaced with three smaller ones and the clients liked it. It provided a chance to read magazines and newspapers in this new layout, and to put their belongings on the table next to them. They were talking, drinking tea and reading some family magazines. Overall, everything was running smoothly, but for a few problems, of course. It was difficult to be across everything. Staff insisted on testing clients' urine samples for traces of drugs. The coordinator asked them to stop and explained the harm reduction nature of our work. Basically, we accepted continued heroin use while minimising the harms until the person was ready to quit. The addiction field had moved on from being punitive and punishing users who provided a urine sample with drugs in it. In fact, we preferred them not to test for drugs. These days staff would examine why the person was still getting stoned when they were in treatment and if they required a higher dose of methadone. Previously, three contaminated urines meant patients were expelled from the program.

The midwife had treated many clients, mostly for gynaecological problems. Initially, she was required to work three days a week but was so inundated with clients wanting to consult her, her days were increased. A few days later, when I asked her if there were any problems, she said the coordinator knew about them. In April 2009, two clients were pregnant. Prior to that one client had reached full term and there had been three or four referrals for abortion. One woman had been pregnant four times and so the midwife gave her a Depo-Provera injection, the contraceptive that lasts three months.

Previously, the midwife's husband was unhappy when she took this job on, but he had come around and was fine with it now. He didn't want her being involved with these people. I guess he meant drug fiends and other undesirables, but I wasn't sure. She asked to receive some training to increase her skills base. She had completed over 150 Pap smear tests.

She received USD220 a month, whereas a researcher received USD550 month. I suppose it didn't help that they docked her salary because she was late one day. The boss didn't pay her superannuation. She didn't want to complain, because these jobs were uncommon in Iran. Later, I heard conflicting reports about paying superannuation. I was unable to decide who to believe. But all the clients adored her. She provided training sessions for the clients on vaginal hygiene, contraception and marital sexual problems. She taught family planning, conducted STI tests and provided contraception. On a typical day, she saw three to five clients. I felt like hugging her.

The lawyer assisted clients with problems related to their families and finances. Within a few weeks she was at ease in her role and had assisted several clients with serious legal matters. One client did not have an ID card, without which she was unable to negotiate any red tape or government departments. An ID card was essential even to rent a hotel room. She gave advice to the clients, but they did not follow her guidance; in fact, they did nothing about their problems. Sometimes there was no improvement, which disappointed her, but she thought some had improved from their attendance. She said 'Those who had quit drugs appeared more presentable.' It was good if the clinic could continue because it was helping clients; they loved it here and thought that this was their home. The director thought one day a week was sufficient time for the lawyer to be here when the social worker followed up the clients.

The psychologist had worked here for nearly two years. She ran individual and group therapy, using a behavioural psychotherapy approach, delivered education and did crisis intervention. She enjoyed her job, even though it was more difficult than working in a private clinic. These clients were more trouble, less motivated and illiterate. Small indicators of progress were evident, but the reason why was a mystery. She believed knowing that there was a place for them here lifted their self-esteem.

The social worker had introduced carpet weaving classes and some general training to improve clients' skills in computing, typing, sewing and candle making. She held weekly educational sessions, where the clients selected the topic for discussion. She had also negotiated with a welfare organisation to provide loans to clients to start a business once they learnt a new skill.

At first the clients were reluctant to take condoms, so the nurses started discussions on how to use them. Clients were given cosmetics as a reward for joining a group on a regular basis. They also provided some basic food such as omelettes, soup and spaghetti for the clients.

I had a meeting with some staff to hear their views on their work and clients.

One said 'I never thought that people who inject heroin could be trusted, but they are just regular people who happen to be deprived of most social and health services that are afforded to everyone else.'

Another said 'It has been quite a journey for me to gain a better insight and understanding of the most disenfranchised part of the society. They have been through all this misery and suffering but are courageous to withstand all this and still be able laugh and care about each other.'

And a third said 'This group deserves the best but instead suffers ignorance and rejection from almost everybody, even health professionals. I admire the level of concern and support that these patients have for each other and their kids when their own lives are difficult.'

But most commented on the poverty experienced by some women and that staff needed training around this.

Our doctor had been with us for nearly a year when we first met. She had a private practice and had worked in the addiction area before. She found the management structure infuriating as there were too many bosses. There were some problems with clients who were unmotivated, still used drugs, left treatment easily, and worst of all came from a low socio-economic status. The drugs included opium, *kerack*, amphetamine, crystal, marijuana and alcohol. Many clients used Ecstasy, but crystal was popular now. As there was no substitute treatment for crystal meth, treatment needed to focus on psychological help. Staff considered imposing a fine for clients who tested positive for crystal meth, but the clients didn't have the money to pay the fine. I suggested a rewards system instead, but when this was tried no one was able to produce three urines free from drugs in a month. After providing one urine sample free of drugs, they received a certificate. After three certificates they earned a present. They would test anyone who appeared intoxicated and hence were more likely to detect positive results. There was some pressure to prescribe benzodiazepines, so I told the doctor about having policy of not prescribing any at all.

Next up, the administrator put forward her views on the services and the clients: 'Some clients are aggressive and behave badly.'

I started to explain that this was perfectly normal behaviour for people with an addiction. Indeed, some of these antics resulted in their incarceration. But she cut me off, retorting that females took more energy to work with than male clients. I inquired as to why and she stated they were more damaged. She mentioned an Iranian researcher who held a similar viewpoint. Then, as she continued, she revealed a deep concern for them as they were more vulnerable to sexual assault than male clients. I should have followed this point to ascertain if she meant they were more vulnerable now and, if so, we should explore some options to reduce it. Then her face lit up as she espoused quite spontaneously that there were a multitude of wonderful aspects to her job. She mentioned the spiritual aspect to it. It was rewarding when a client improved, and she felt that they had contributed to this. And this, she beamed, was a daily experience for her.

There was no process by which a complaint could be raised without the whistle-blower being singled out. I suggested that a client representative might meet with management to raise any concerns. Other complaints concerned restricted access to the toilet, forcing some to venture to a public toilet in a nearby park. This could dissuade them from staying and having informal chats with the staff. Even the client with the bladder problem who often wet herself had to scoot across to the park. I raised these concerns with the staff and asked about the toilet and if clients could use it and was told some clients could use the toilet if they were not using drugs, but other clients had put rubbish down it and blocked it. So access for everyone was not possible.

Soon all women would be required to pay USD15 a month for their methadone treatment, which, up until now, had been free for them. Even so they still had the better deal as the men were paying up to USD70 a month for their methadone. Men were allowed takeaway doses, whereas the women weren't. But I couldn't see how this depended on payment.

Next the criticisms focused on being dosed the correct amount of methadone. A few sceptics believed that part of their dose of methadone was missing, and that they went into withdrawals as a result. Worse still was the underlying assumption that the staff were creaming off some methadone for some monetary gain, possibly selling it on the black market. I refused to pursue this line of thought with these impressionable down and outs. Instead I calmly made light of the comment by revealing we hear the identical concerns back in Sydney and invited them to consider the coincidence of that. Nevertheless, I raised these concerns with the clinical director later, and he reassured me that the dispensing of the methadone was accurate. He religiously checked the records himself and confirmed that there were no discrepancies with methadone dosage.

The coordinator was due to have a caesarean section and sent one final report. There were 53 clients, of whom two were new. But they came for just two days and then disappeared. As soon as we drew some into our place, they drifted away and obviously it would be a challenge to find out why after they had gone. I told her we could cover her maternity leave so she could stay home with her baby for a few months. Somehow this was misinterpreted as she has been sacked and several phone calls were required to sort it. I sent a brightly coloured blanket for her son and managed to post it before she gave birth. She was quite chuffed with it and the fact that it came from the other side of the world. She showed it to me when I next visited, and it looked well loved.

A quick chat with those who hadn't drifted away revealed some reasons why their peers had. One woman was admitted to hospital, one was expelled for dealing drugs and a third client found the distance to reach us was too great. Another woman's husband was imprisoned, and yet another had migrated. Also, some clients were referred to a service closer to them, but finally and perhaps most disturbing was the woman who left because she was struggling with staff.

Back in the safe room a new focus group was about to start. Several of us sat in a circle, in anticipation of our next discussion topic. New clients were a little shy about opening up to us, while the old hands were experts in critiquing the arrangement of the room, the staff's manners and even the food provided. Everyone began by praising the staff. It was important for the staff to hear these compliments about their work. The old hands were making a good use of the services and felt at ease with the staff. Some who had drifted away had tried to go cold turkey or abruptly stop using methadone but resumed using heroin or opium. One young girl said this was the first time she had been able to stay off heroin for several weeks, while others nodded in agreement. Another woman said it was easier this time with the support that we had offered them. The topic meandered around until I wondered aloud if a separate space was essential, separate from the men.

Another said 'Yes, of course—we don't want men around when we see the doctor or the nurse.'

Being able to remove their hejabs was not a reason, but being with peers and being away from men were though.

The next time I sat in the safe room I was with a different interpreter, Mitra. We just chatted with the several occupants. There appeared to be a regular crowd who came and hung out in the safe room. Again, the conversation turned to money. All these complaints were about having insufficient money. One patient had several sons who along with her husband were all addicts and in methadone treatment. She complained that soon she would have to pay for her treatment. Clients predicted that they would have to commit a crime, if a fee was introduced.

So a female-only service was deemed important. It encouraged them to while away their days here, so they felt at ease and had better access to the services. Most were shunned when visiting doctors in the community, so understandably they welcomed the chance to consult one each and every day and free of charge.

One woman said 'That is what I like best about the place, being able to ask the doctor about my problems when I want and without being hurried out of the surgery.'

People who used drugs were notorious for doctor shopping, which is where they go from one to another to procure different drugs from them. I had discussed this behaviour with our doctor and asked if she found clients pestered her to prescribe medications like sleeping pills? When she said yes, I suggested a blanket ban on this if it was out of hand. That was what some centres did in Sydney: they put a sign up that said NO SLEEPING PILLS WILL BE PRESCRIBED HERE.

Then the gripes came bubbling up. Maryam whinged 'I don't like the opening hours; to arrive on time is difficult for me.'

Our hours were from 8 am to 3 pm for women and then from 3 pm onwards it was for men. If a woman came later, she could receive her methadone, but all the dedicated workers were gone and the place was inundated with male drug users.

She continued, 'When I missed three days in a row, I was kicked off the program and I don't think that's fair.'

Actually, what happened was that a client's dose was gradually reduced and then she was taken off the program. If they were not turning up, it's a sure thing they were using heroin again. So it was official policy and a safety measure. I tried to explain this to her but she wasn't going to listen.

At this point, the nurses and doctor were shuffled out of the room.

Once again, I found myself alone with females without any staff being present. The first time I was in Evin Prison hearing their complaints; I hadn't really followed through there with the woes of those incarcerated, apart from mentioning one or two to the prison director who seemed familiar with issues. But now, I had some responsibility for the services on offer. The clients couldn't wait to open up about their problems with the staff, their men folk and the world. My interpreter moved her chair closer to mine, which I read as a sign of support. She had prepared me for some of the complaints, but other complaints seemed to be quite serious breaches of protocol that needed investigating. A secretary, who happened to be a psychologist, was dispensing methadone to clients. Even though she did the job well, this was against the rules, even in Iran. This "stand-in-nurse" knew the clients by name and she had a good rapport with them, but still it was against the rules.

I had to raise my concern about this practise. Just one wrong move could cause untold problems for us; we could lose our licence to operate as a methadone service, leaving hundreds of clients, female and male, without treatment.

Another focus group was held and this time I had come to listen to their thoughts on the staff in their absence. 'Anyone want to say something?' I asked the group. Several hands went up followed by statements that they didn't like the rules; there were too many rules. I explained that the workers didn't make the rules; they just enforced them. Most of the rules were the same at all the methadone units in Iran—in the world in fact. But this piece of information was irrelevant to those who were preoccupied with a major health problem like drug addiction. The dislike of homeless clients was a worry, as it might be driving some users away from seeking help.

'I don't like them, the homeless—they should go somewhere else,' one client stated.

I was left wondering what the stigma was about being homeless. One of my researchers had been raising the issue but I had not paid it much attention, until now.

Fariba told us she travelled to the Caspian Sea for the New Year with her husband and child and returned exclaiming that her holiday was superb. It was the first time she wasn't bothered searching for drugs. The period of celebrating New Year in Iran can carry on for 13 days. The first few days were spent visiting relatives and exchanging gifts. On the last Tuesday of the year, *Chahar Shanbeh Suri*, people go onto the streets to light small bonfires and jump over them shouting 'give me your beautiful red colour. Take my sickly pallor away.' They believe that by passing over the fire, all their illnesses and misfortunes will disappear. The children race onto the streets banging pots and pans with spoons to chase out the last Wednesday of the year. Then they go knocking on people's doors to ask for offerings. The New Year tradition sees Iranians buying clothes and cleaning their houses. A *Haftsin* table is set that holds seven items all beginning with the Persian letter "S". Wheat or barley symbolises rebirth, a sweet pudding symbolises affluence, dried fruit and garlic represent love and medicine, apples represent beauty and health, sumac the sunrise and vinegar symbolises old age and patience. On the last day of the *Nowruz*, New Year celebrations, people leave their homes to picnic in parks. The New Year had fallen just a month before my visit in April. Iran has a different calendar to the West. They use the Solar *Hejri* calendar. So their New Year starts on March 21st and is a celebration of spring Equinox. Also, we started in 2007, which was actually 1388 in the Iranian calendar. This year denotes Muhammad's migration from Mecca to Medina, rather than the birth of Christ, which was the start date in the Western or Gregorian calendar.

Two clients had applied to go away for the New Year holiday. They wanted a few days' doses at once, but it was against the rules. If they missed a day, withdrawals would start. Some clients had not returned to us after the New Year holidays. The manager thought those who had not returned might re appear, but the doctor thought they had moved away. The missing clients were a concern as their absence signalled one thing: they were back on heroin.

Work marched on at the clinic. About a dozen clients were chatting, eating and drinking tea and, of course, smoking cigarettes in the safe room. Two days earlier it was the birthday of one of the clients' children, and they had a small celebration in the safe room. I worried about children coming along when school was on.

The psychologist attended a training course about psychosocial treatments for addiction, but she had to pay. She learnt many things, but really we should have paid for her to attend. One of the nurses and one of the secretaries who was a psychologist went on a counselling course. I questioned why the secretary attended these courses, when anyone of several other staffers could have gone. There seemed to be some nepotism going on. Staff dealing with the clients needed to attend these courses, I suggested to them.

Today there were 48 clients, of whom five were brand new. As usual, some clients were in the safe room, eating, drinking, talking and fossicking. I asked why were they always searching their bags? They were looking for any remnants of drugs, loose change, and food even. The doctor had a new job in another city and would leave us in six weeks. So we had to cajole another doctor into working with us. Not many doctors want drug users as their patients, as they can be difficult, always demanding more of this, more of that, trying to procure sleeping pills and the like. However, I liked the challenge of working with them. Most have just had it tough; nearly all have been sexually or emotionally abused.

It was now the month of *Bahman*, 21st January to 19th February, 2010. The director complained that the rent had risen by 30% and there were other costs to be met, like staff training. The cost of methadone, the core treatment, would rise by 15%. He also said that the midwife who was working two days a week would have her time increased to four days a week because of the need. These extra days would cost USD150 a week. I couldn't see how we could move money around as the budget was so tight. The scholarships we had planned had to be cancelled, as the funding for my research centre had been halved.

Now it was *Khordad*, the next month, and 94 women had registered. But this success was tempered by the departure of 44 souls. The coordinator had returned after a break of six weeks following the birth of her son. She noted that the new doctor was fitting in well; she was active and interested in her job. Although she was new to the field of addiction, she wanted to learn from the doctor in the men's clinic. She would undergo some training as soon as possible. The new doctor was worried about clients who continued using drugs while on methadone, especially one who was three months' pregnant. As she was new to treatment, her dose was still low and was not maintaining her yet. It would be increased at a steady rate. But in the meantime she was using opium occasionally to stave off the withdrawals.

One client who was a hairdresser was assisted to set up a hair salon in one of the rooms. The room was minimal; just a table with a mirror on it and a chair in front of it. Glamourous women with big hairs dos looked down from the posters on the wall. On the windowsill sat bottles to spray water. I assumed the hairdresser had brought her scissors when she came as I couldn't see any implements there. There were a few other ornaments around to give the impression of a salon such as magazines, hairbrushes and clips. She would cut and colour clients' hair for a small fee once a week. We funded the supplies for it. This add-on was popular with clients and attracted more clients to the centre. The social worker felt that this helped bring about a change in attitude in the clients, and that they felt better about themselves. One had to worry, though—if there was a fight, would the scissors be used to sort an argument? The more I observed the women, the more often bad behaviour came to the fore.

It was time to inform key people in the field about our efforts. A four-hour advisory meeting with stakeholders was planned with a free lunch for 20 people. Several staff members made presentations and the guests were invited to ask questions. And they did. They wanted to know who was the funder, what were the clients like and what were the rules for being expelled. They all wanted to know what services were on offer and the composition of staff.

The software for data entry had been installed and piloted on the first 20 clients and found to be working fine. It was a bonus to access data quickly. We were able to share that our clients' use of stimulants had abated just a little. Unfortunately, it was not due our work; rather the police had arrested stimulant dealers on the streets. The psychologist and the social worker would attend a workshop about stimulant use to learn how to manage those who use the drug. The dealers would be back. And the clients would use stimulants again.

Today, the doctor had 46 clients on her books, which was a hefty case load for a rather inexperienced doctor, considering most were damaged individuals. The psychologist tried to attract more clients to her groups by hosting sessions on family problems, and interpersonal issues, but no one was turning up. The midwife did a routine check-up for all the clients, and even visited a few at home. The social worker had clients making statues and doing textiles. It was a hive of activity for the staff, at least. But some event had deterred a few women from participating. Even in the safe room, three women just sat there staring into space. The TV was on, but they were not watching it. When they were asked if there was a problem, they said they didn't like the new rules. They could drink tea at specific times only. Smoking was prohibited and there were no more hot meals.

I couldn't see the sense in stopping these things as they had been the draw cards for many clients. Practically everyone drank tea all day long and virtually every user smoked cigarettes. The hot meal was also a hook. The coordinator asked me to see what instigated the change. Most offices in Iran have a waitress who serves tea and fruit, constantly. I was a bit confused when they sent the first bill, which included a fee for a waitress. The waitress had surgery a few days ago and was unable to cook the meals for the staff and clients. Some clients thought that other clients were informing the staff about their dealings, so they didn't feel comfortable. This could have been in part due to the personality traits of drug users.

I asked the director if perhaps there was another room where they could smoke cigarettes. And why couldn't they have a cuppa whenever they liked? He told me when the waitress has recovered there would be hot meals again. But he seemed to ignore my other concerns.

Many of my earlier visits had focused on problems for those imprisoned, the staff and the clients. This was the time to listen to some solutions, some successes and be convinced that at least some women had commenced their recovery. Today's group discussion was just that: how were they faring? One young girl said she was better off financially as she wasn't wasting all her money on drugs. Another said she secured a job and could now pay off her debts. I remember hearing about this girl who had a job, they were so rare that you could count them on one finger. Bijan had told me they made a special arrangement so she could collect her methadone earlier than everyone else in order to be at work on time. She didn't want to have to disclose her addiction to her boss as why she would be late for work. She was sure he would fire her.

The door swung open with a bang as a scruffy woman pushed her way into the interview room, sat down and interrupted our discussion. Maryam gestured for the woman to go ahead with her news. The intruder wore a green shirt and a pale yellow hejab, with a small hole in it. Her conversation was deliberate and directed at me. She smiled and continued chatting away for the several minutes it took for the interpreter to remind me who she was. Apparently, I gave her a keyring last year, but I still couldn't place her. She was intent on speaking, so we listened. As her story was being interpreted, I began to recognise her. She was the homeless girl, Fariba, the one whose story brought tears to my eyes, whenever I retold it. The change in her hair colour had confused me. Fariba was a brunette before and now she was blonde. Her journey into drugs began at 14 with opium, when her friend gave her some heroin, for free. The poor girl had been incarcerated more than 20 times, she has slept on the streets, been beaten by her brothers and her father. She first came here seven years ago. Then I understood she just wanted to inform me that she was here and willing to be interviewed.

Maryam resumed control of the discussion and continued her story. 'My mother died while giving birth to me. I was the youngest. With no one to care for me and my siblings, dad brought us to Tehran and placed us in an orphanage. Then my uncle, who was childless, accepted me as his baby. After six years, my uncle's wife had a child and his wife's attitude changed towards me. Sometimes they beat me, but they never abused me sexually. But I had a good relationship with my cousins. They were like my brothers and sisters. I loved my uncle but not my aunt. I didn't know my uncle wasn't my dad and was astonished to learn this secret.'

On she went. 'During 2nd Grade, my uncle told me to stop calling him dad. I was just eight years old. I fell behind at school, failing exams because my world was shattered. I had to repeat 2nd Grade twice. Most of my uncle's attention was directed towards his own kids. My aunt made me marry a 40-year-old man when I was 14 years old. I resisted but felt I had no choice. My real father visited me, but he had no concern for me and even years later when we met again.'

At 14, Maryam was under the legal age for marriage, so she was his temporary wife for three years. She lived with him, but he was a loner and could not relate well with others. She felt alone. She hated that man. When she was 17, they married legally. On her wedding night she became pregnant, but her aunt was jealous and wouldn't take her to hospital when she was in labour. Her uncle helped her with the baby, but it died when she was three months old; it was sick and premature. Then Maryam had a second baby, but this strained her marriage, so she divorced with the support of her neighbours. After that, she moved into her brother's home, but his wife demanded he kick her out or she would leave. Maryam overheard this ultimatum while dozing. It was a squeeze in the house with three people living in just one room. Maryam's anger was directed at her family for arranging her marriage, which she believed led to all her troubles.

By the age of 18, Maryam tried her hand at factory work, making clothes. Her ex-husband took the baby with him, which she agreed to as she didn't have a place for even herself. Her ex-husband didn't marry for nine years as he longed to be a couple again, but Maryam refused. Unbeknownst to Maryam, when she rented a room, it was in the same building as a brothel. The madam in charge smoked opium and Maryam's only social outlet was to join her. She knew naught about opium and had no idea she could become addicted.

After the Islamic revolution in 1979, the brothel that Maryam lived in was demolished with a wrecking ball. Luckily, she was evicted just prior to its destruction. Seventy men and 70 women who were connected with the brothel were hanged at Tehran prison, the very prison I visited on my first trip, and the one I was trying to visit again. She was taken to prison to view the executions. After they were executed, they were shot in the head and their families were required to pay for the cost of the bullet. She felt a sense of relief as she thought they deserved to be executed as they were selling sex and drugs and had evicted her for not participating. She wasn't executed as a witness came forward to swear that she was not involved in unlawful activities in the brothel and that she was an addict. Although she did not escape being punished completely; she received 100 lashes and a two-year prison sentence.

On her release from prison, no one came to collect her so she was shipped out to a welfare centre. There they gave her a room and a job working in a day care centre. She received USD4 a month and a loan of USD30, which was a substantial amount back then. She was very satisfied with their help as they looked after her. But Maryam continued her friendship with addicts so was asked to leave the welfare centre, and then she rented a room and worked as a cleaner. About this time, she was introduced to her current husband who was 20 years her senior and they married. Parviz, her husband, was a musician with irregular work. Her friend told Parviz that Maryam had a problem; just opium not heroin, but the truth was the exact opposite. Parviz accepted her and promised to help her quit. Once married, she did manage to quit heroin but then returned to opium. About six to seven years ago a friend told her about methadone, and she ventured into the Persepolis Centre where she has remained, partly as she was afraid to stop.

Maryam confessed that she smoked crystal meth last year, as well as taking Ritalin, a stimulant to treat attention deficit disorder. Maryam's neighbours were *kerack* users but brought some crystal over and provided Parviz with a customary free sample. Parviz and Maryam spent that night and the next day smoking it in a pipe. Within hours Maryam was sweating excessively, restless, suffering a migraine and experiencing palpitations—and swore she would never smoke crystal again. Her resolve, to abstain, was strong again. It was rather difficult to believe that was the only time she dabbled in other drugs while in treatment, or that she would not succumb again, but she was adamant. Her husband still ate opium and was a client at the main clinic.

*

Long days of wearing a hejab had flattened my hair, which was overdue for a trim. A friend recommended a salon and promptly took me to visit. The salon was above one flight of marble stairs in an upmarket mall in North Tehran. After opening an ordinary looking door, we were confronted by a hefty tapestry curtain that shielded the internal operations from prying eyes. Inside the ant colony-like salon, glamorous types seemed to glide around tending to their charges' hair. All heads swivelled to focus on me. I slowly took off my coat and hejab and wondered what they were thinking. A young trainee took my coat to hang up and escorted me to a chair. As I turned to thank my chaperone, it was only then I realised she had left me to play out my desired hair cut like a game of charades.

As the room returned to normal, I was asked if I spoke Farsi, or Arabic or surely French, no? Embarrassingly I shook my head for each language and tentatively offered English. Another young girl was summonsed to discuss my intended haircut. My plan was to have a minor adjustment to the length, but the lady had a different idea. The next few moments were spent on the customary questions about how was my family, where was I from, what did my husband do and how many children did I have?

'Tsk tsk' was my hairdresser's response to my reply of no husband. And so the charade of began of how my hair needed more off the sides than the back. I was fascinated to observe the lady in the neighbouring chair having her errant hairs removed by threading, the twisting of two threads quickly together and rolling them across her chin. Meanwhile, my attending lady snipped away and soon I was ushered to the counter to pay and left the beehive of activity. I donned my hejab and coat and off I went back to the streets of North Tehran.

Chapter 10. Back to Iran

In February 2009, another chance to visit Iran came when I was invited to present our results at Iran's National Drug Conference. I had sent my passport to the Iranian Embassy in January but when it hadn't been processed, I decided to drive to Canberra to obtain the visa in person. I was reminded of Bijan driving the length of Iran to secure his visa to travel to the Slovenian Conference, where we first met. Then an official from the Iranian Embassy rang to say 'your visa is ready, just present your passport and complete a form agreeing to abide by our laws.' The drive to Canberra was a six-hour round trip. My mum came along as company—just like Bijan's father-in-law had accompanied him. I also had to make an emergency visit to the dentist and then travel onto Sydney for another hour and half to catch the plane, all in one day. I left Monday night, two weeks later than planned. Originally, I was timing my trip to coincide with Easter, which meant my mum can mind my twins and I wouldn't skip too much work at my office. But that coincided with the Iranian New Year period; a holiday of 13 days. One colleague in Iran asked 'Can you postpone the trip for a few weeks? No one will be at work.'

One pressing issue to resolve was the non-payment of the coordinator's salary for a month a while ago. I had about six dinner dates already. One new friend wanted me to come dinner at her place, but it was the night the Conference dinner was scheduled. I asked if the two events were close to each other, which might allow me to attend both in one night. With so much of my energy devoted to the clinic and the women, I felt their daily highs and lows. Yet being on the other side of the world, communicating only via phone or email was no substitute for being there.

Effat, a friend in Tehran, was set on me to staying with her—and her newborn twins. But to have a holiday from my own twins and a chance to catch up on some sleep was too tempting, so I booked a hotel room. She kept pushing me. 'My kids are not that noisy. Anyway, I'm not sure what kind of hotel the Taj Mahal is. OK, you can stay there one night if you want some sleep, but I can't let you stay there if it is in a cheap street. You must stay with me. My place has a traditional toilet, but Hussein is going to buy a Western one for your comfort.' She kept berating me. 'I will pick up you from airport. Tell me the flight number and the time it arrives in Tehran; tell me the Tehran time.'

I had been calling her husband Abdul Hussein, which was his name, but I found out much later it was impolite of me to call him that. I should have addressed him as Mr. Hussein because of the (slight) age difference. My friend didn't seem to mind; in fact, she laughed about it. It took another friend to point out my error. He was very depressed when he was in Australia; he wasn't suited to being a house-husband. But when I called on him at home in Iran with his new twin girls, he was bursting with delight.

I disembarked the plane at Imam Khomeini International Airport in Tehran at 10 pm and was met by Effat, her husband, her twins and a nephew. She waved across the hall, summonsing me to walk around the security, but I waited in line. I had brought a twin pram for her as she couldn't find one in Iran. She had been a magnificent friend when I had my twins. She actually showed me how to breastfeed. And insisted I stay longer in hospital to feel comfortable with caring for my babies. We all climbed into a small car without seat belts or baby capsules. I was very concerned because the Iranians are erratic drivers and seemed to ignore the road rules.

During that visit I saw three car crashes. One crash may have resulted in a serious injury, if not death. A truck had crashed into the back of a car, mounting it and squashing it flat. Then there was a fire on the road. This accident was on the way to the airport as I was leaving. I kept asking my driver to slow down, but he couldn't understand me. I was terrified as we sped along way over the 120 km/hr limit. More than 20,000 Iranians die in car crashes every year.

I acquiesced and stayed with her the first night but I desperately wanted to stay in a hotel so I could sleep and come and go as I pleased. My hotel, the Taj Mahal, was in North Tehran. It had an Indian restaurant downstairs where I ate my breakfast and met the coordinator before we would set off on the hour's journey to South Tehran. I'd have a plain breakfast, *lavash* with some *tabrizi,* a white cheese and occasionally *haleem* and a cup of stewed coffee. The other options were too spicy for my bland palate. Over breakfast, the coordinator and I would plan our mission for the day ahead; who to meet, what issues to tackle and if there any particular clients to catch up with that day. The poor coordinator was over her job; she had resigned but still accompanied me to ensure I witnessed certain aspects. The hour's drive gave us time to gossip, to catch up on each other's kids. We had been emailing and ringing each other for three years, so it was good to meet in person again.

I asked if I could take off my hejab in the car and she says 'Are you crazy? If the police see you, they will put you in jail.'

We both laughed as I had asked her several times how could I visit prison this time. I wanted to observe the prison methadone unit and interview any women I was following if they were detained there.

The clinic had moved to new premises about a year ago and that meant some clients didn't move with them. They had told them several times and in different ways, but they didn't make the move. Some might have been imprisoned. This trip was the time to determine whether they were improving, in terms of their use of substances. If the treatment was effective, then we should know. Other aspects of their lives would fall into line, like their ability to function socially, their depression and their risky behaviour in terms of drugs and sex should all change for the better.

Clients were asked if they had an infection like HIV or Hepatitis C and whether they were willing be tested for these infections, once soon after they arrived and again after about six months. If the therapy was working, new cases of infections would be rare. If someone had been infected, we could treat it, especially if it was a sexually transmissible infection. If some had HIV or Hepatitis C infection, we would have to refer them on to a specialist.

When I asked the director about his thoughts on the service, he commented that it was a harm reduction service for females that had achieved many its objectives. But then on he went to list problems. Again, he said the position of lawyer was not so useful; he and the clients preferred a psychiatrist. It wasn't personal but there were limitations on what she could do for clients. He had no problems with any of the staff. The social worker was an expert in her area. Her bad temper was due to taking on too many duties; I thought she should reduce her hours. I asked about the claim that she dosed the clients with methadone, but he said she never dosed clients with methadone or determined their dose. He held weekly meetings with staff in groups and on an individual basis. Their main gripe was to have more leave as they only received two days per month. Nor did he have any problems with clients, just with managing the staff.

The discussions with my colleague in Poland raised some concerns for us. We were both funding the same organisation and wondered if there was some double dipping happening. We had external and independent accountants for our respective projects. She had also encountered trouble transferring funding and routed their funds through Germany and France. He said 90% of their funds came from abroad. Elsewhere methadone was USD80 a month for men and USD40 for females. Here was it USD70 a month for men and free for our group, but soon they might have to pay. He was not worried about receiving foreign money, as long as it didn't come from the USA.

Our research had been presented in Beirut, Barcelona, Arizona and Florida, but by other people so far. This was the first time I would present our data. I felt a real sense of achievement explaining our findings which had come to fruition after seven long years.

At conferences, researchers can either present their work with a ten-minute oral presentation or they can display a large poster on a board with details of their work. We received an oral presentation. But it appeared we had chosen to report on a week with a low level of activity. The coordinator told me 'pick another week, one that shows how busy we were with them.' My presentations gave the opportunity to tell others of the lessons we had learned while running our project. One staff member wanted to mention the resistance we had faced in the neighbourhood and how we overcame it. Several neighbours did not want such an agency in their midst. Another staff member said 'Let's inform everyone how beneficial it was to have a midwife or lawyer on hand.'

Actually, it benefited the homeless immensely to have free access to these professionals. Clients were asked for their input as to what should be in the presentation. One woman said 'Since coming here I have saved money to buy milk and nappies for my baby, which I couldn't do when I was using drugs.' Another one told us 'I have started sewing clothes at home and I am earning money, legally. I don't spend any money on heroin. Finally, I feel like a mother for the first time in my life.' She beamed.

All these little bits and pieces were channelled into making a wonderful talk for the conference, which attracted a lot of attention from the attendees. I attended the conference; ideally, a female staff member would have attended, but no one was proficient enough in English to answer questions that might arise. The coordinator would have been the obvious choice, but she was unable to attend as she had a new born.

Rumours were that methadone bloats your tummy and rots your teeth. It would take time to debunk some of these myths. Some were worried that it would be more of a battle to come off methadone than it was to come off heroin or opium. But what they didn't understand was that they had to transfer to methadone to get off heroin or opium. I reassured them that we would ask the doctor to repeat the session explaining methadone and its side effects. She would talk about how long they should stay on methadone, the interpreter explained. They were happy with this and all nodded in agreement. Then the coordinator pointed how this was the first experience for many in their recovery from drugs.

During the month of Farvardin, which runs from the 20th of March to 19th of April, the social worker had eight clients crocheting and knitting. The plan was to make dolls that could be sold to earn some pocket money. When I visited another agency, they were knitting similar dolls. Somehow, I was persuaded to buy all the dolls that had been made, over 20 dolls, each costing USD3. I needed a magician's suitcase to squeeze them all inside. So I positioned them around my hotel room to provide some company for the next hotel guest.

This visit allowed another follow up on the progress of several women, including Zahra. I wondered what the outcome was for her baby, and for her. I put my questions to several staff, but no one seemed to know. I pestered them to quiz other clients if they had any knowledge. For several days, I hassled them to discover what was her fate. What about the service where her husband was—did they know what had become of her? If they found her, could they encourage her to come back and talk to me again? She had stopped on a pinnacle. Did she tumble into some crevice or did she manage to come down off the mountain without any injury?

According to our most recent information, she was determined to leave methadone behind. Some time elapsed leaving me to surmise they were unable to locate Zahra or any information about her. Then at lunch one day in the staff room, the administrator came in and made a comment to the interpreter who reacted as if she had just been bitten by a snake. The interpreter said they found Zahra. She had the baby, but it had been stillborn. She was very depressed and shunned treatment. The air was heavy. We had failed her and her baby. What could we have done differently to have prevented this tragedy? Everyone around the table was a mother: me with twins, the coordinator with her boy and the administrator due to give birth to her second baby. We all felt her loss as a mother.

When we started our clinic, another one was about to open at roughly the same time. In the intervening four years, another three clinics for females struggling with drugs have opened in Tehran. When I delivered one training workshop, I requested that staff from another service be invited. They came along but didn't stay afterwards to mingle. Attempts to encourage our staff to meet the other workers were to no avail. One training session was on females who use drugs and AIDS or HIV to be precise, and the other was on reproductive health. I was up at 3am preparing for them.

I was fortunate enough to call on another centre, again accompanied by my interpreter. This centre had moved into new premises that seemed much more welcoming. I recognized the director immediately and we hugged. An official from the UN was visiting at the same time, so I trailed behind him. As we were in the foyer a fight broke out in a Narcotics Anonymous meeting. The one who came off worse from the fight was put in a room where she whimpered a bit and held her hand. We had heard about this meeting and how it was closed to non-users. So, when we were offered a chance to look in, I declined. We did see the methadone dispensing area. A few familiar faces from the other clinic were waving at us as they recognized us. We saw the vocational training room and I bought a few knitted dolls and discussed the possibility of doing some research with their clients. They had a small room for children of clients with some toys in it. We came just before lunch and saw the cook heating up some cans of tuna to mix in a rice dish. One client had drawn a series of disturbing pictures revealing her dismay with life.

*

Another season had past, and winter was upon us. We asked Mona to join us for another focus group discussion. She was still rolling up daily, so she must have been sorting her life out and improving some more. While this sounded encouraging, Mona's appearance had deteriorated in several ways. Her makeup was looking tired and again there was that whiff of poor hygiene. I suspected Mona had switched to using stimulants, probably crystal methamphetamines, but I did not have a chance to ask as she spoke at a telegraphic pace. She had abstained from heroin for seven months and, according to her, didn't have a severe heroin problem—no craving. But she had acquired an addiction to crystal meth. Although Mona wasn't living with users, she passed her time with them. Later that week, her urine sample had traces of amphetamines and narcotics. Mona was using crystal meth and heroin. She then asked about what treatment was there for crystal users. When she stopped using crystal, she had nightmares and became suicidal, so her husband sourced some more crystal. Someone suggested checking into a medicated detoxification unit with cognitive behavioural therapy. She just shrugged. Her recovery was one step forward, two steps to the side and then three steps backwards.

Mona spoke with some authority on the drug scene, another indication she was back on the gear. 'The more expensive the drug, the stronger it will be', she declared before nodding off. Either her dose of methadone was too high or more likely she had topped up with some heroin today. Meanwhile the others chatted about sex. After a few minutes she woke up to inform us that 'sex workers in North Tehran use condoms but not the ones in South Tehran. They don't use them'. I asked 'how come they take condoms from us in South Tehran?' She seemed not to hear my question and drifted off again into her narcotic haze.

One is exposed to infections when one shares a needle to take drugs. When clients had been enrolled for some time, it was appropriate to discussing these various infections. In general, most agreed to have a test for HIV infection and all the results came back negative. I was so relieved. We had established the service before the HIV epidemic had taken hold. But when I compared the interview schedules to the serology, I realized some HIV positive persons had declined to be tested. Whether the infection was the result of sex or drugs, no one knew, not even them I suspected. Our researcher had told me about the stigma HIV positive people faced and now it was becoming apparent.

HIV was not the only infection we tested; we also investigated the level of Hepatitis C infection and transmission. More patients tested positive for Hepatitis C than knew they had the infection. While four reported having been infected with Hepatitis C, eight women had tested positive, exactly double the number. It was almost certainly due injecting drugs with shared syringes. Yet quite a few had been adamant that they had never used a syringe to take drugs, but their test results told another story. I decided to explore these discrepancies of serology and self-reported results.

Mona's serology indicated she had managed to avoid HIV infection, again. But as she was clearly relieved to hear this result, I was left thinking perhaps there was a risky event where she might have been exposed.

'My husband doesn't use drugs and my family doesn't know I use drugs,' she said.

I just nodded, but all the while thinking you are fooling yourself, my dear. Somehow, she had convinced herself of this. It would take some time for her to face up to reality, a prerequisite to recover fully from her addiction. Apparently, her mother died recently and when she had requested several takeaway doses to enable her to attend the funeral in another town, she was refused. Some office gossip suggested that her mother had died three times already.

Then Mona stopped attending suddenly. Our staff was unsure what had become of her. I pestered a staff member to canvass other clients who knew her outside. The news was terrible. Her crystal meth habit had taken hold rendering her psychotic. She suffered outbursts of violence and extreme anxiety, which forced her husband to move her into the garage in the basement of their building. He was attempting to have her committed to a psychiatric hospital. He blamed the crystal meth for sending her crazy. Yet he had been so violent, she sent her child to stay with relatives far away.

For the third time the possibility of hiring a psychiatrist was raised. The hourly wage was just USD14. Imagine so many years of study to be a psychiatrist for such a modest salary. The plan was to employ a female psychiatrist for four hours a week during which, if she saw two clients an hour that would be eight a week. During *Esfand*, the last month of the Iranian year, the search for a psychiatrist began. A request was made to reach out to Mona and invite her back to be one of the first clients of the psychiatrist, if she hadn't been scheduled.

I was keen to know whether there had been any improvement in their involvement in crime. It was low at the beginning; just three women dealt drugs and one committed a violent crime before coming to treatment. After a few months in treatment, only one was dealing drugs but yet six said they committed a violent crime in the last month. These were small numbers, too small to see if there had been any significant change. Those crimes were probably related to crystal use.

One area where there was a clear improvement was in how well they functioned socially. The number who reported being employed had increased and by a significant amount. Fewer clients were living with others who used drugs, which would help them recover. The second area was anxiety; many users had a reduced level of anxiety. There was some lifting of depression when we repeated the Beck Depression Inventory and some improvement in their somatic symptoms. We requested urine samples to test for the presence of substances, indicating recent use. Early on three women tested positive for heroin and after a few months six provided positive samples. One person acquired Hepatitis C during the period between her two interviews, but luckily no one acquired HIV infection. At the start, all were diagnosed as dependent but after a few months only one quarter met the criteria. So we were treating addiction, to heroin at least.

Fariba proudly declared all her problems had been blown away, like cobwebs off a tree. And she wondered aloud 'what kind of job can I have? I can't read but I could learn to sew. Can I learn that here?'

Her behaviour appeared like a regular person's, well, at least one in recovery from addiction. Was she mentally ready to work? I asked the social worker, who shook her head and pursed her lips. She said 'Maybe when Avat is enrolled in school. Also, much work remained to be done with her husband and the reasons for her staying out late at night'. I asked 'Why was she doing that?'

The social worker shrugged her shoulders and smirked, indicating that Fariba was probably playing up in some way or other. The administrator came in, poured herself a cup of tea, and added her considered view on Fariba. 'I'm not convinced that she has recovered. Recovery does not flow like a river but rather it lurches from a flood to a drought.'

These girls binged for weeks at a time then halted completely and resolutely. Surely Fariba had gained some traction against her habit? The administrator relented, there might some improvements but staying out late and still using crystal would cause problems for her, her marriage and little Avat. She was failing. The administrator and the social worker agreed. The administrator foresaw that when they began to charge for methadone, as planned in a few months, Fariba would leave.

It was time to try a slightly different tact. Was there anything that could be addressed for her? The interpreter said 'well, she still has a few problems with a reoccurring urinary tract infection.'

I was sure the midwife had tried to treat her with antibiotics. Maybe she needed to see a specialist? I asked the interpreter could we refer her to a specialist for that problem. But that would cost money. I said 'OK, let's see if we could find the money to cover her treatment and ask the midwife to take her to the specialist.' In my mind this woman was a definite success story. But the real question was how long would she be required to attend. If she stopped coming, she would return to using within a matter of days, if not hours. The clinic was her life now, so we needed to fill her life with things like work or study to keep her from gravitating to drugs. I asked the staff about encouraging her to enrol in a class; maybe she could learn to read and write, like her daughter was about to.

Maryam said 'my friends and family can see a positive change, and they are so pleased for me. My kids are so glad I'm at home cooking *ash* (a thick soup) for them, and my friends are relieved I'm not trying to borrow money off them.' And my daughter said I look like her mum again.'

She went on to say she could relate somewhat better to her husband and was no longer throwing things at him—which drew a number of laughs from the circle—and her friends had stopped shunning her. Everyone was talking to each other and her family was more welcoming of her now she was rebuilding her life. She had been very depressed, bordering on suicide but now she felt upbeat about her future.

*

My host escorted me to a bazaar one night. It was so alive, with a soccer match on TV and men calling to each other across the narrow alleyways about the game. We stumbled upon a café and rested for a while. The waitress inquired as to what had brought me here. For once, I just wanted to say I'm a tourist, but I would still have to justify that response. In an average week I might spot four tourists in Tehran. Instead, I admitted to doing some work with the UN, skipping over the minor details of addiction, which allowed her to smile and nod.

Next, we slipped into a shop that seemed to be from yesteryear. Piles of rugs on the floor nearly reached the ceiling, forcing the shopkeeper to climb a ladder to peel back layers of deep red carpets. Small wooden boxes with inlays sat in cabinets; some were for tissues, some were for pencils. As I started to make a mound of items to buy, the shopkeeper offered me a cup of tea and ordered a young boy to fetch a chair.

We strolled along the alleys in the bazaar under the soaring crypt like ceilings. A spice stall had heaped mounds of mustard, red and white coloured spices in opened hessian bags. The copper pot stall was fringed with pans hanging from the door frame. Light beams rained down through the gaps in the roof illuminating the dusty air. It was cold outside, so I preferred to be in here where it was cosy. It was sprinkling when we came in. But it was tomb-like inside with no signs of what the outside world was like. Then she drove me back at my hotel which surprised me as I thought she had said come for dinner. Then it was too late to eat at the restaurant and I wasn't game to walk around the neighbourhood looking for a kebab. So I turned in for the night, without dinner.

The following evening, the coordinator hosted me at her house to meet her husband and child, which I gladly accepted, but insisted on buying take away food so as to avoid cooking. She would be tired, working and looking after her young baby. She over ordered and we didn't eat until quite late. She was busy with her baby who was still up way past 10 pm. I was so tempted to offer some advice about establishing a routine for the baby but also knew she must sort it out for herself, just like the clinic workers must sort out how to do their job. New mothers always fuss too much over their first born and then ease back a bit when the second one comes along—although when I had two at once, I didn't have time to fuss. I didn't even have time to do up all the buttons on their clothes or even change mine. In the early days, it took three hours to feed and change them and they needed feeding every four hours! I would go to sleep in my clothes for the next day, so when I awoke, I was dressed for the day. If I was still in my pyjamas at midday, I felt like a failure. We sat up so late that I was nearly asleep before dinner was served. She was complaining about the superintendent in the building who wouldn't let them put up a satellite dish.

I excused myself as I had to call it a night. My hotel room was like a small apartment, with a kitchen, lounge room and a separate bedroom. And the mini bar was free. There was a TV and I was hooked on the local channel. I couldn't understand most of it but it was interesting to watch. I also enjoyed reading the local English language newspaper. There had been something like 300 visits between Iraq and Iran in the previous year, which seemed pretty impressive in terms of cooperation. Iran had also donated much funding to Afghanistan for some humanitarian project. These activities didn't make the news back home.

Another night I was invited to dinner by my host and this was where the earlier confusion was. She was house sitting her parents' house as hers was being painted. I wanted to take a small contribution for the dinner, but obviously I couldn't take wine, the normal offering in Australia. So I wandered down the street from my hotel to buy some fruit or sweets.

The shopkeeper was surprised to see me. I can hardly speak any Farsi, so I had to point to things, which was fine until I wanted a small box instead of a bag for the fruit. For a few minutes I tried to indicate this with my hands until finally I saw an empty box and pointed to it. He nodded and rushed to retrieve it. He then offered me two boxes, though I only wanted one.

On the way back to the hotel I saw a commotion on the road. I wasn't quite sure what it was at first and, without thinking, I just asked someone what happened. He said it was a car crash and they were arguing over whose fault it was, in perfect English. He was taken aback with me being there.

At my hotel two workers were always ready to bale me up for a chat. A lady on reception had a huge bandage across her nose. I found out later that nearly everyone was having a rhinoplasty procedure in Iran. The bell boy was studying public health and had many questions about my work. He had heard of our service and was eager to visit with me. Unfortunately, it didn't seem appropriate to take him into their sanctuary. So I told him stories from my daily trips there.

At dinner that night several others were also invited. There was a couple who were in same line of work and a colleague of the host and his wife. I had met his wife on her trip to Sydney where I was able to show her around the red-light area of Sydney and the gay quarter. Her area of expertise was sexuality, so I knew those areas would interest her. At first, I heard she couldn't make the dinner, then, when she turned up, I was surprised at how happy I was to meet a friend.

That night we had so much ground to cover. One guy was a senior researcher, yet he was quite playful and very, very funny. He asked me how things were working out. I had to tread carefully as I knew they would have heard of some problems but at the same time I didn't want to be too critical as we were achieving many goals. Over 240 women had come through the doors and for most it was their first attempt at beating addiction. I highlighted the research, which was the real draw card of our project, with him being a researcher.

Another colleague of mine took me to dinner twice at the most famous restaurant in Tehran. He was my hero. He was very instrumental in introducing harm reduction in Iran. He told me a funny story where his wife was so upset, he took her to the doctor, even though he was doctor. After a few minutes the doctor called him in and said his wife was upset because he was a workaholic. I had met his lovely wife and made a point of telling her how important her husband's work had been, not just for Iran but for many other countries. Being a hero in your own country can be hard, let alone your own home.

One Thursday, my host accompanied me to Tehran's Museum of Contemporary Art. On the way there we passed a guy creating figures out of twisted wire to sell. The figures were about six cm high and had some musical instrument or other object to show the figure's trade or hobby. We stopped to chat, and he asked what had brought me here. 'Training workers about harm reduction and HIV,' I told him. Immediately he opened up about his past problem with heroin and how he was fine as he was in Narcotics Anonymous. He was chain-smoking, though. I asked him whether he found it hard to stay clean, and he said as long as he had a task to busy himself with, he was all right, but when he was bored, he got tempted to use again. He also said he needed to earn money to stay out of trouble.

Once I looked at him, I could see the tell-tale signs of his past, but I hadn't noticed it when we stopped. I was pleased as this meant I must be off duty. Meanwhile, a school bus filled with kids pulled up beside us and all the kids pointed and laughed at my hejab. It was different but not that funny. Once inside the museum we encountered more children who were a bit older, but they were laughing at me as well.

The museum has a winding ramp snaking up the inside of the building. I couldn't wait to visit the shop and buy some books and postcards. It was said to have the largest collection of valuable Western modern art outside Europe and the US, but I was interested in viewing the Iranian art.

I appreciated the time to socialise with my friend in a relaxed environment. We chatted about politics, art, religion and the weather as two friends might. We stopped for a drink and funnily enough they didn't have any coke or cola in the cafe, so I settled for a juice. It was stifling hot, yet it had been snowing earlier that day. The hejab and *Roopoosh*, were very uncomfortable on hot days.

There were a few other people in the cafe and the worker serving behind the counter inquired as to my reason for being in their country. Again, I was asked for my thoughts on their country. My experience of the country was somewhat skewed. I wondered if I should say I found the prostitutes very charming and the prisoners on death row pleasant, but actually it was the drug-addicted women I had come to visit.

Later that week, Effat and I strolled along the street with her twins in the pram. We passed by some men sitting on a wall. One old guy asked where I was from. 'Australia,' I offered. Then another one confided that his brother had just died in the devastating bush fires that had recently ravished one state back home. Almost two hundred people died in the fires in February 2009. We stopped for a short while, offered our condolences and had a photo taken with them. It seemed very strange to have had a connection with this man on the streets of North Tehran.

*

As the clinic had moved, Bijan requested to be sent many photos of the new premises. There were six or seven patients I was desperately seeking, but most had drifted away from our project. Finally, I heard that the staff had located some. But I was unable to excuse myself from running several workshops for staff. I also wanted visit two other agencies. It was so satisfying to know two more agencies dedicated to help women struggling with these problems had opened up.

Apparently, two women I was desperately seeking had been imprisoned, and I began to wonder if I could visit them. I made requests to my colleagues about accessing the prison. But a UN staffer says she couldn't visit prison for her projects and didn't think I would be able to either. I approached another colleague who suggested writing to the deputy at prison and asking her. He introduced us by email and asked her, but I didn't hear anything back. After a few days I emailed her directly. She answered that if they had not committed a serious crime or a political crime, I might be able to visit and interview them. I was fairly certain they would have committed just petty crimes. I sent her my list of several patients and said that, although I had heard two were in prison, I didn't know which two. Believing that if I could show I knew two were in prison, she wouldn't think I was just trying my luck. I had promised to inquire only about their time in the community with us, in particular, and nothing about prison. I stressed I was willing for a guard to be present for the interviews to ensure the discussion was limited to what I had promised.

*

Previously, our presentations of work had focused on improvements in heroin using behaviour, but this time I detailed clients' sexual behaviour and improvements. I began with a comparison of female to male users, drawing on the international literature, as very little was known about female drug users in Iran. It was known that females started using drugs later than males but sought help sooner. Of course, what really differentiated them were their relationships. Females tended to have partners who also used heroin, whereas males didn't because there were five, six or even ten male users for every female user. Men were the usually the ones who initiated their partner into drug use; mostly it was the boyfriends or husbands but occasionally it was the sons or fathers. Females with drug problems were more likely to have a mental illness than males.

I felt I had to explain how I came to be there, what my involvement was, how I met Bijan in 2002 and visited Iranian prisons where I saw poor wretched souls needing assistance not punishment. Also, I had to cover what we aimed to do, to set up a centre for those in Evin Prison. We had such grand plans to provide free methadone treatment, sexual health care, a needle and syringe program, primary healthcare, counselling, employment training, a lawyer to help with their legal problems, and finally, a space where they could just be—a safe room.

Although Bijan and I had met back then, it took another four years to secure the funding and one more year before we opened in 2007.[7] We had decided to place the women's clinic in the general Persepolis Clinic, which had a few female clients. It was crucial that we employed a range of female staff to make them feel at ease. The key person would be the doctor, at least in our minds, but actually it was the midwife who was appreciated the most. Her role included offering Pap smear tests, advice on family planning and screening and treating sexually transmissible infections.

The doctor was necessary for primary health care and assessments for methadone treatment. She was assisted by two nurses who dosed the patients and also provided the harm reduction service of a distributing

---

[7] Dolan et al., 2011b.

needles and syringes and condoms. While this might have seemed a trivial issue, the combination of treatment and harm reduction was quite a sticking point for many service providers. I remember when we opened the needle and syringe program in Australia. Our program was next door to a methadone unit and one of their workers kept tearing down my sign, which informed people that they could collect free syringes from us.

While methadone was a useful aid for many patients, they also needed the psychologist to address issues such as the "addictive personality" and craving. They were taught parenting skills; an essential element, if their mistakes were not to be inherited by the next generation.

The high hopes we harboured for our lawyer and the work she would do were dashed somewhat. A few problems like securing ID cards and issues surrounding custody of children were resolved. But she was unable or unwilling to assist Mona with her divorce. She did educate them about their rights, but, as the director told me, the law favours the man in Iran, and it was a waste having a lawyer when they preferred to have a psychiatrist. We tried to employ one but we were unable to. After determining how depressed our women were, I could see why this kind of assistance was so desperately warranted. The idea of the safe room, a women-only room happened but again not as I had imagined. I thought they would come in and remove their hejabs, but I was the only one to do so. I guessed once they have put them on, they leave them on for the day.

The social worker was a key player at the service, with many ideas even helping one woman set up a hair salon inside. She was concerned about their welfare and visited them at home, prompting me to be concerned about her safety. She was intent on improving their vocational skills, though to be honest most women were unable to work at any meaningful task. As she summed it up, the major goal was to empower women. They wanted to work but there were no job openings for them as people rarely accepted them. The stigma was debilitating for them. She ran some workshops to show them how to do handicrafts, but they were slow and tired easily. They were pretty lazy, if we were to be honest.

The results from the research were very favourable. Amazingly over 240 women had climbed the dingy stairs of our building looking for help. Although only 97 had registered during the study period, nearly all agreed to an in-depth interview. We had to explore their behaviour before they came here and more importantly how they behaved during their stint in treatment. We managed to interview 60 and re-interview 40 or so some months after their first interview.[8] My favourite activity was the focus groups where we delved into their lives; their childhoods, their marriages, their relationships with their children and their journey into this drug scene. Interviewing each staff member was illuminating for me to hear their thoughts, feelings and suggestions.

One client was a sex worker but was unwilling to admit it. I surmised she didn't feel comfortable disclosing this to the staff. Was there a problem with confidentiality or a judgmental response? This was one area where we didn't achieve as much as we had wanted. I had planned to help establish a peer group for sex workers, like we had in Sydney, but of course that was not possible. The social worker proudly told me there were ten clients who engaged in sex work the previous year. It was very important, she told me, that they practiced safe sex. But this sounded like she was more worried about the clients of sex workers than the workers themselves. She said they kept their confidence, but I was not convinced. I had wanted transsexuals to be able to use our service too, but they didn't come. I did meet two transsexuals on my last trip, but they were too frightened to attend.

But the thing no one could predict was how common and severe depression was among these women. One hundred per cent were classified as depressed and over eighty per cent were severely or moderately depressed. It is incredibly tough to change your behaviour when you're depressed, but yet many managed some behavioural change.

---

[8] Dolan et al., 2012.

Chapter 11. Making a Difference

The clinic was located in a heavy heroin using area, Shoosh Square. Normally, my coordinator accompanied me to the clinic but one day I had tried to get a taxi there on my own. Even though I had been there many times, I still couldn't find it. The taxi driver kept circling the intersection, but I couldn't see where I had to go. In the end I had to ring a friend and ask her to direct the driver over my mobile to where I wanted to go. I had walked around the area a bit and must admit I felt a bit uneasy. Not because I thought something would happen to me but, rather, I attracted a few strange looks because it was obvious from my attire that I was not a local. The traffic in Tehran was crazy. The city was huge with scant attention paid to road rules. I was struck by how many people hitchhiked. Cars slowed down, the driver called out where he was headed and, if the destination suited someone, they jumped in. I was startled when women jumped in cars with men in them. It kind of reminded me of street walkers plying their trade to men who were kerb crawling. There was however a distinct separation of the sexes on the buses. Men rode up the front while women were relegated to the back. The sexes were segregated on the metro, too, with women only in carriages and mixed carriages.

When we reinterviewed the women, we knew about some of issues they were up against, even before we talked to them. For example, some had drifted away, some had left town, but of concern were that two women had been admitted to psychiatric hospital. One had mania and the other had a schizophrenic diagnosis. Another two had been imprisoned. Just keeping them sane and out of prison would be a constant challenge. Often stopping amphetamines use can impact upon one's mental health. Stopping amphetamines use would usually remedy one's psychosis.

I asked again if they could help Mona with her divorce. They claimed she hadn't told the whole truth. I felt I had to support the staff and side with them, if there were conflicting stories. People who use drugs face many legal problems. However, if we were to continue with this project, the director told me again he preferred to have a psychiatrist on staff rather than a lawyer.

The management of clients was the social worker's job. She had tried to show clients how to make dresses but they couldn't be bothered to learn. We were about to wind up the research side of the project, so I wondering if we still needed a coordinator. The director stated we didn't need one for these last two months but if we did another project we would.

That evening at my hotel, my interpreter and I waited for the lady from the UN to take us to a women's refuge. She came to my hotel and ordered tea thinking we would take some time but we were ready. I kept insisting to my interpreter that she did not have to accompany me as we had been together day and night for three days now. She had a husband and son, but my protesting was in vain. So off the three of us ventured to South Tehran stopping to buy some dates, sanitary pads and sweets from a Northern town called *Kloocheh*.

Our destination was a refuge but the windy streets without signs proved challenging, so around and around we drove in dark, narrow alleys for a while. The streets were dirty and the buildings were run down and old. It was very different from North Tehran. I felt uncomfortable with taxi driver who was to take us home. I was sitting in the front and felt vulnerable. We finally located the refuge and walked down a very narrow alley. As we entered, I could smell gas and tried to raise an alarm, but someone said that was the developing world for you. We sat in the office and chatted and listened to the work being undertaken. Some clients sat around too. All workers at this refuge were ex-clients. They were being forced out of the building by the landlord as the neighbours complained that the women dressed up and wore makeup, which was code for being a sex worker. Two girls sat in the corner hugging each other.

As we removed our hejabs in the office, we heard of the many problems with the neighbours, some even came to protest in the middle of the night. There was much noise when the girls were stoned, calling out to men, taunting them. The mayor wanted the refuge moved to the outskirts of the city, but the need was here. They were searching for another building on the main street perhaps—the UN lady promised to arrange a meeting with the mayor.

Children were prohibited from this service. A mother had to give up her child to the State to be allowed to stay here. Women could arrive after 3 pm and stay until 9 am the next day. Services include bathing facilities, 30 beds, breakfast and laundry. During the cold months, the service is full. In the warmer months, it's half-full as clients who want to use drugs stay on the streets. This particular night it wasn't too cold, so there were about eight or ten women inside. Drugs were prohibited inside. Staff searched clients' bags for any contraband. The sleeping arrangements reflected the drug-using status of the residents; non-users slept in one room and users in another room. It was somewhat revealing that the non-users' room contained four beds, while the users' room had 26 beds. Basically, the refuge catered for those who were addicted but allowed those who were abstinent to stay as well.

The kitchen was down a few very steep steps, halfway below ground level. My interpreter commented that this was a typical house with the kitchen and the cooking duties hidden away. The showers were down there too. Fish was on the menu that night. We were invited to join them for dinner, and I was keen to do so. But my interpreter insisted we had something on, dinner actually. On the other side of the open-air courtyard was the current users' room. The council wanted them to put a roof on the courtyard in case a neighbour could see in, but no one could since there were no overlooking buildings under the starless sky. Some were complaining about not having a completely separate space for those who wanting to quit, explaining it was unsatisfactory to stay at the same place as those who were still using drugs.

In the users' room we had the chance to chat with the women. One worker asked what I wanted to ask them, but I couldn't think of anything at that point. They all looked damaged and had had a tough time, not just of late but for most of their life. Then a worker said let's ask them if they want to say anything. I was reminded of my visit to Evin Prison some 10 years earlier, and how we decided then to help them, which started me on my own incredible voyage.

A few minor complaints came first; the beds were uncomfortable as the mattresses were too thin. The wire bed-base looked terribly uncomfortable. Another mentioned that they didn't have television or music. Then one lady pleaded that she needed an operation, a hysterectomy, and therefore some financial assistance. Another had cataracts and required an operation on her eyes to prevent glaucoma. A tall resident who was young and spoke excellent English was there with her mother who had the eye problem. She had learnt English when living in the USA and Brazil for some time and had come back Iran to be with her mother but had become addicted, like her mother.

Another resident lamented that her daughter was in Mashhad, 900 km away, so they could meet only every six months. Her daughter had been given over to the State. The lady in charge started to cry, then, like dominoes, each woman around the circle started to cry, including me. I quizzed the UN lady if there was anything we could do. Her priority was to meet with the mayor to ensure the service continued to operate, and not be run out of town.

When we were leaving the lady in charge gave me a strong hug; we knew the challenges these women were facing and felt solidarity doing this kind of work.

*

On my last day at the clinic, as soon as I entered the safe room, a slender well-attired woman crossed the room and walked directly towards me. Was this a new worker I was yet to meet? Her makeup was understated; her lips a slight crimson colour revealing bright healthy teeth. Her skin looked alive and well cared for and her clothes were smart. On her wrist she had an expensive looking watch and a mobile phone hung around her neck.

The interpreter relayed what she was saying as she approached me. 'I have been coming here for four years now.'

I was still unsure as to who she was as I couldn't recognise her. She grabbed me tight around my forearms. I couldn't read her mind—was she about to clonk me on the head? Instead, she kissed me bang on the lips and said 'I love you, I love you, I love you. You have saved my life.'

All I could think about was what kind of infections can you get from kissing? And the inclination to wipe my mouth was almost impossible to resist. She hugged me so tight I could barely breathe. And then she pinched my cheek, hard and we both laughed. I knew then it was Maryam. She was unrecognisable, at least to me.

Grabbing my hands in hers, she escorted me over to a bench like we were old friends about to catch up on each other's news. She regaled story after story to me without worrying about the interpreter who I was motioning to come over and join us. The interpreter put her hand on my shoulder, 'You can tell her life is wonderful again.' But how, I wondered. What had changed? I wanted details.

Maryam looked radiant; the weight lost made her look younger and fresher. Maryam wasn't hankering for money, nor was she using drugs. It was plain to see. She prohibited all use of drugs in her home, which was in sharp contrast to her previous life where she hung out with 25 users a day, though it was unclear if those gatherings were in her house or elsewhere. She raised her finger and slowly stated 'There is no socializing with others who use; I do this to keep safe.'

All the benchmarks of a heavily dependent user's life had dissipated; she wasn't turning any tricks, committing any crime, hadn't been hospitalised and hadn't overdosed for years. In sharp contrast, when she first came along, she was overdosing on a weekly basis. The poor old dear had been trapped in her intoxicated cocoon for 33 years. She was one of the first through the door, having been a client when the main clinic was overrun with men. For virtually every day for the last four years, she had turned up to drink her methadone.

Maryam's relationship with her daughter and grandchild was healthy and she was even at ease with Parviz, too. Her main supporter and confidant was a cousin who covered the cost of her treatment. For too many years, Maryam had no contact with her daughter who was unable to finish school because Maryam was absent. Her life, now, was problem-free. She was very content to stay home, although her arthritis probably stopped her from taking any manual jobs. But I wondered if she was too old to be gainfully employed. Being illiterate and having a long history of heroin abuse would limit Maryam's job options. I gave her a tea towel with some Australian animals on it. She laughed and said she was still using the tea towel from an earlier trip!

She declared that she was cured; without any problems, cravings or withdrawal symptoms. The essence of her life had changed. I had to know who she lived with as I remembered she had lived in a house full of users. I suspected that she had been a dealer, but I never knew for certain.

The interpreter said 'She lives by herself, and it was something she had to do to be drug free again.'

'What else?' I asked the interpreter to ask her. It almost seemed as if the details didn't matter to either of them, just to me. She was in recovery and that was that.

'She gets along well with her family, her friends and even her husband.' the interpreter said.

At that point a few girls laughed about this comment as they had heard her complain about her husband for years. Her cousin had stuck by her all these years, apparently never using herself. At times the friendship was definitely strained. She had to leave as she had a date with her friend to go shopping at the market and have a cup of tea.

Epilogue

Epilogue

Our women's-only clinic has since closed with most of the women transferring to the Persepolis main clinic. With more women in attendance, it will be less threatening and more welcoming for them. It was very expensive to provide the boutique service we had provided. There is still a place for women-only services, or at least women-only sessions in mixed clinics.

Sustainability is a key goal in international development. While it will not always be possible to continue specialised clinics like this one, it is often hoped that the main stream services can change to accommodate minority groups who need specific services.

129

References

Day, C. Nassirimanesh, B. Shakeshaft, A. & Dolan, K. Patterns of drug use among a sample of drug users and injecting drug users attending a GP clinic in Iran. *Harm Reduction Journal 3*:2 doi:10.1186/1477-7517-3-2, 2006.

Dolan, K. Hall, W. & Wodak, A. Evidence of HIV transmission in an Australian Prison. Letter. *Med J Aust*, 1994;160;11:734.

Dolan, K. Salimi, S. Nassirimanesh, B. Mohsenifar, S. & Mokri, A. The establishment of a methadone treatment clinic for women in Tehran, Iran. *J Public Health Policy*, 2011a, 32, 219–230. doi:10.1057/jphp.2011.10.

Dolan, K. Salimi, S. Nassirimanesh, B. Mohsenifar, S. Allsop, D. & Mokri, A. Characteristics of Iranian women seeking drug treatment. *J Womens Health* (Larchmt). 2011b; 20(11):1687–1691.

Dolan, K. Salimi, S. Nassirimanesh, B. Mohsenifar, S. Allsop, D. & Mokri, A. Six-month follow-up of Iranian women in methadone treatment: drug use, social functioning, crime, and HIV and HCV seroincidence. *Substance Abuse and Rehabilitation* 2012:3 (Suppl 1) 37-43.

Shakeshaft, A. Nassirimanesh, B. Day, C. & Dolan, K. Perceptions of substance use, treatment options and training needs among Iranian primary care physicians. *International Journal for Equity in Health*, 2005; 4:7. doi:10.1186/1475-9276-4-7.

Turnbull, PJ. Stimson, GV. & Dolan, KA. Prevalence of HIV infection among ex-prisoners in England. *Brit Med J*, 1992; 304:90-91.

Wodak, A. Dolan, K. Imrie, A. Gold, J. Wolk, J. Whyte, B. & Cooper, D. Antibodies to the human immunodeficiency virus in needles and syringes used by intravenous drug abusers. *Med J Aust*, 1987; 147:275-276.

www.ingramcontent.com/pod-product-compliance
Lightning Source LLC
Chambersburg PA
CBHW070924270326
41927CB00011B/2719